T0286350

OWN YOUR THRONE

HOW TO MAKE YOUR TIME IN THE LOO WORK FOR YOU

BRADFORD WARE

Illustrations by Em Spitler

CHRONICLE BOOKS

SAN FRANCISCO

Library of Congress Cataloging-in-Publication Data is available.

ISBN 978-1-7972-2265-3

Manufactured in China.

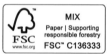

MIX
Paper | Supporting responsible forestry
FSC™ C136333

Design by Evelyn Furuta.

10 9 8 7 6 5 4 3 2 1

Chronicle books and gifts are available at special quantity discounts to corporations, professional associations, literacy programs, and other organizations. For details and discount information, please contact our premiums department at corporatesales@chroniclebooks.com or at 1-800-759-0190.

Chronicle Books LLC
680 Second Street
San Francisco, California 94107
www.chroniclebooks.com

CONTENTS

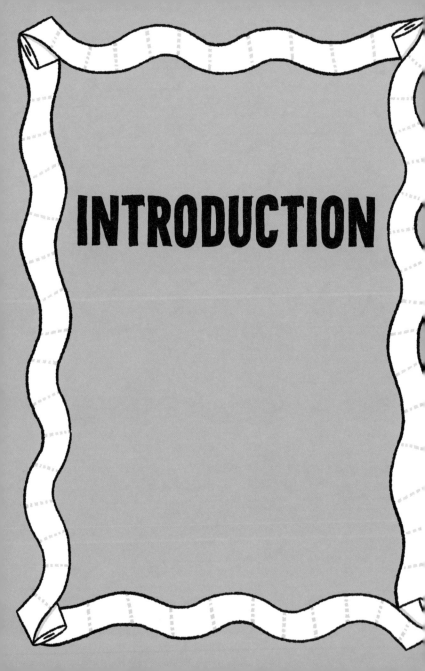

INTRODUCTION

COME TAKE A SEAT

I have no idea where you are right now.[1] But I know where you'll eventually be going. Maybe in a couple minutes, or a few hours, but I am absolutely confident there is a visit to the toilet in your not-too-distant future.

Nature can call at any time, and it's typically not a call you can ignore.[2] It calls in the middle of a first date, half-way through a job interview, or during an afternoon run. Answering that inevitable call may be an uneventful journey for some—or at least that's what they say—but for many honest folks, that journey can be a significant challenge that's bravely faced every day. Some even battle through multiple rounds. But even the bathroom champions among us never get the recognition we deserve. We just wake up the next morning and do it all over again.

The truth is, nearly 40 percent of adults worldwide suffer from functional gastrointestinal disorders, so almost half of our population could be considered "power users" of the bathroom. Even if you just (conservatively) spend fifteen minutes on the toilet every day, that's more than three hundred days

---

1   Wait, are you in a bookstore? Wow! What section was I in? Oh, by the way, this book contains footnotes.
2   Possibly the most annoying butt dial.

over an eighty-year lifetime—**almost a full year of your life**. Time is precious. And I'm here to tell you that nothing should stop you from enjoying every minute of it.

And who am I to say? Honestly . . . nobody, or maybe everybody? I'm just a normal person who uses the toilet like everyone else on this planet. But if titles and credentials really matter to you, then, yes, I am technically an expert.

Malcolm Gladwell popularly stated that you need around ten thousand hours—roughly ten years—of experience in a field to become an expert. Since I regularly eat ice cream and pizza despite having an extremely cranky bowel, I probably hit the ten-thousand-hour mark every year.

I've struggled on toilets my whole life. And even though I've suffered more than enough flare-ups of over-wiping wrist strain,[3] I refuse to give up quesadillas, or having a chocolate malt milkshake with my fries, so I've officially accepted the side effects of my condition. But that doesn't mean I suffer. On the contrary: I enjoy the food I love, and I've learned how to really enjoy my daily time on the toilet. And I want to share that battle-tested knowledge with you—and to help you discover a unique formula for *your* perfect toilet experience.

So I don't want you to change your diet to try to reduce your time in the bathroom—actually, quite the opposite. Let's instead embrace and enjoy our time on the toilet just like a

---

3   It doesn't get as much media attention as tennis elbow, but I assure you it's just as serious.

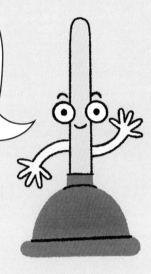

Hi, I'm Plungie! I noticed that you are reading a book about toilets! I am here to help answer some of the deep questions that are common to most of us (but we might feel silly or afraid to ask) so that everyone can go like a pro. Never fear—Plungie is here!

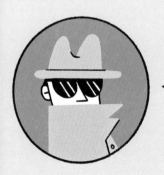

FBI (Federal Bathroom Investigator) Agent 002 here, from this toilet team. Throughout the book I'll occasionally offer you missions. Should you choose to accept them, these field activities will require you to defuse some tricky situations with tactical toilet responses.

great meal—because each experience comes in all shapes and sizes. Let's take some time to understand why sometimes you leave the bathroom feeling relieved, and other times feeling stressed. There are so many factors that can make a toilet customer feel dissatisfied, satisfied, or even pleasantly surprised. From my experiences as a loyal toilet customer for over 30 years—across this country and others, from hotel lobbies to rest stops to porta-potties and, yes, even a few bidets—I can help you feel prepared and confident for whatever toilet situations lie ahead, such as:

- Finding the best restroom on a road trip
- Dealing with a clogged toilet in a sticky situation
- Using a "customers only" toilet without buying something
- Choosing the right stall for your circumstances
- Going beyond toilet paper into the world of bidets
- Surviving when your only option is nature's toilet

So take a literal bathroom break with me and learn all about upgrading your time on the throne. Because in the end, we don't choose our bathroom journey—it very much chooses us. But it doesn't have to be like taking the ring to Mordor; the experience can and should be enjoyable. Nature is calling—answer it. Make every throne your very own.

PERFECT TOILET EXPERIENCE FORMULA

Big Bathroom doesn't want you to know this, but there is in fact a secret formula[4] for having the perfect toilet experience. The *Perception of Our Potties* (POOP) equation takes in several inputs related to the bathroom experience and outputs a *Pleasantness Objective Output* (POO) figure, like a credit score for toilets. Many variables are at play that can turn a pooper's paradise into a defecator's disaster, so it's imperative to keep these factors in mind when you are squatting.

$$\text{POO RATING} = \frac{(D_{oo})(N\Omega t^4)}{[(C_L \infty G)^{Ir}] \, X}$$

- D_{oo} = Turd Type. This is the state of the actual poop; they come in a variety of forms with unique potential complications that change on a meal-by-meal basis.
- N = Noise (Ambient). The louder the room, the less potential for your booty music to be heard.

---

4   Doesn't quite have the historical clout of other formulas like the Pythagorean theorem, but I promise it'll be more useful in your everyday life.

- Ω = Outfit Coefficient. What are you wearing and how easily can it be shed? This is the intersection of fashion and function.
- t^4 = Time, Temperature, Traffic, and Toilet Specs (Big Four). Are you in a rush? Is this bathroom particularly warm[5] or unnecessarily chilly? How many people are coming and going? Does *your* seat fit on the seat?
- C_L = Cleanliness Constant. Includes everything from scent to sinks, and, yes, most definitely the seat too.
- ∞ = Random Chaos Infinity. We all know restroom experiences are anything but predictable. It's not a mistake that this has an infinite value either.
- G = Grossness Threshold. Can be described as the immediate NO thought after laying eyes on a toilet candidate. More a feeling than a mathematical value, the tolerance for grossness level varies greatly from person to person (see next formula factor).
- I = Individual (You). Your unique preferences, time on toilet mood, and in-the-moment emotions. Our baggage doesn't stop at the bathroom door.
- Γ = Gamma, Desperation Score. How thankful and relieved are you that you finally found this bathroom? What's the nearby restroom quality? A fast-food restroom in a sea of porta-potties can feel like Buckingham Palace.

---

5   This can be a huge driver of Sweaty Butt Syndrome (SBS).

- X = The X Factor. This variable encompasses all the intangibles of a bathroom experience. What are those exactly? Gotta keep reading!

TOILET TYPES

Let's begin with the basics, like the first week of school where you review everything you learned last year. Here are the fundamental toilets, also known as the *Big Five of the Bathroom Industry*. You've seen them all before, and you've experienced their various advantages and disadvantages IRL.

HOME

Tried and true, the headquarters for your hindquarters. You should feel a strong connection when you settle your double moons into its well-worn saddle. It's my hope that you create a strong connection with your home toilet, just like in the movie *Avatar* where the Na'vi (Pandora natives) bond with the Banshees (flying bird-things) before riding them. Your partner-in-crime in taming your colon.

Pros: Familiar, private (hopefully), safe (really hopefully), customizable, convenient, clean

Cons: If you have to share it with someone who doesn't respect better bathrooming philosophy

STANDALONE/SINGLE USER

The Great Value version of your home toilet, a lucky find when out and about. Great if you need a power nap or just a general break from the world.

Pros: Four walls of security, spacious, private, also got diaper-changing station

Cons: Can be a bit stressful during restroom rush hour if people are waiting outside

STALLS

The Toilet of the People, found in every school, park, gym, workplace, transit hub. They come in all shapes and sizes, so choose wisely (see p. 24, Stall Selection).

Pros: Industrial-grade toilets, interesting graffiti, others to blame for your bathroom noise, jumbo-size toilet paper rolls—use as much as you want!

Cons: The toilet paper may actually be sandpaper, smell, minimal privacy, the risk of making awkward eye contact through the gap between the door and the wall, and you're never quite alone when sitting on this throne.

PORTA-POTTIES

As the name suggests these portable toilets bring the bathroom to you, established in places where plumbing hasn't yet found market penetration. Originally created during WWII for crews working on loading docks.

Pros: You're alone, and you're not pooping on the ground.

Cons: Flushing technology has never seemed so advanced and underappreciated. If you didn't have claustrophobia when you walked in, you will when you leave.

BIDETS

Considered the premier bathroom experience: a hands-free, no-wiping encounter!

Pros: Toilet paper is completely obsolete; cleanliness can be more thorough.

Cons: These bad boys can come with a bunch of buttons, so you need to know how to use them.

TOILET USER TYPES

Users of the toilets (us) also have types. Find yours and your loved one's below!

- **Quickies:** You don't even notice when they are gone.
- **Slow & Steady:** Go on a regular basis, in every sense. No theatrics or drama—their digestive system is on a strict nine to five.
- **Announcers:** No mystery here. They tell everyone in the room what they are about to do, possibly also

predicting how it will go. Status report to follow on their return.

- **Pig Pen:** Water puddles and footprints on the floor, smudge marks on the mirror, general detritus.
- **Leave No Tracers:** Bathroom is potentially even cleaner after they used it than it was before. More to come on this principle. This is every host's favorite guest.
- **Knockers:** These folks can't come to terms that someone else might already be in the bathroom when they need to go. Will commonly stopwatch your time length when waiting and passive-aggressively announce it when you come back out.
- **Trigger-Happy:** Flush no less than three times every encounter. A Knocker's worst nightmare because they think the person is finished, but it was just another intermediate decoy flush. Experts at avoiding a clogged toilet, but not water friendly in droughts.
- **Group Goer:** Always rallies a squad to hit the stalls together; it's pretty obvious when this person went because half the group is missing. If the party ever becomes boring in the big room, it's a clear sign to hit the bathroom when this person can't be found.

- **Brew Master:** Has a particular scent and always leaves it as their calling card. The aroma of the room should be a clear giveaway here.
- **Hermits:** These users are in for the long haul. They have shut the door on the world, found their happy, quiet place in the bathroom space, and are in no hurry to dispel the magic.

> *Always go to the bathroom when you have the chance.*
> —King George V
>
> *No matter how busy and important you think you are, you cannot reject nature's call.*
> —Michael Bassey Johnson
>
> *Success is like toilet paper: It only seems important when you don't have it.*
> —Richard Jeni

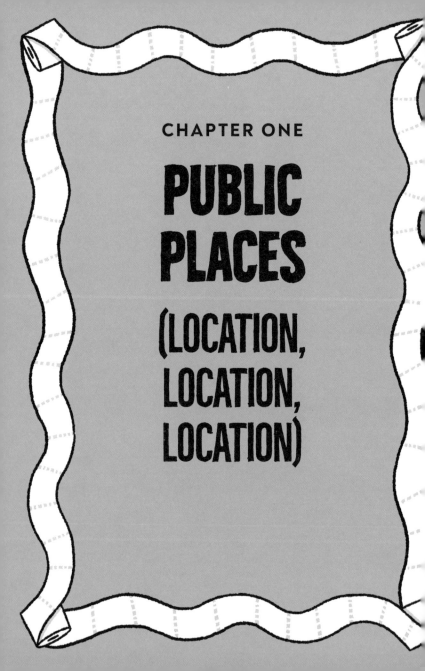

CHAPTER ONE

PUBLIC PLACES

(LOCATION, LOCATION, LOCATION)

OUT AND ABOUT

One of the largest factors for determining the value of a piece of property is its location. This happens to also be the strongest ingredient that impacts our toilet time—where we are when nature calls our mobile line. Some toilets have a view, some have a long line, and others feel like you just entered the Upside Down of *Stranger Things*.[6] While some commode users strive to completely avoid certain toilet situations, I believe you must embrace all cases and be prepared for them, because nature's call can be unpredictable and unforgiving. This book has you covered, whether you are visiting an unfamiliar city, at work or at school, or at someone else's house. Public restroom availability can unfortunately be a substantial problem for folks on the go. A New York City–funded report estimated in 2019 that it had a ratio of just sixteen restrooms per one hundred thousand inhabitants for its 8.5 million population (also the largest population density in the United States). London has very slightly more, with an estimated 1,500 public loos for 8 million inhabitants, according to a 2022 study (NYC's tally is about 1,360). This doesn't

---

6   The toilet situation in the Upside Down was a deleted scene for the Blu-ray limited release.

even factor in that, especially in big cities, public restrooms can be hard to find, have long lines, may be less than clean, and sometimes even cost money. Here's how to find the most comfortable bathroom setups in public settings.

CHOOSING YOUR OWN ADVENTURE: FINDING FACILITIES

When out and about, the most difficult factor in finding a toilet is that you are in unfamiliar territory. Being behind enemy lines is also stressful when you have multiple options. Museums, businesses, restaurants, libraries, shops, transportation hubs, and department stores can be found around every corner in a major city.[7] Each toilet is a different adventure, and it's up to you to decide. So where should you sit?

TECHNOLOGY ENTERS THE CHAT

First, you need to figure out all possible options in your area, and the best way to do that is actually already in your hand. There are now reliable toilet-finding apps[8] available to assist with your search. If you're of the opinion that you already have too many apps downloaded on your phone, map and review apps are also solid options that you probably already have. You can literally put "bathrooms

---

7   Except when they are "Out of Order." Seeing that sign is the most frustrating situation to be in (besides trying to order an ice cream at the McDonald's counter).

8   Technology has finally disrupted the toilet industry.

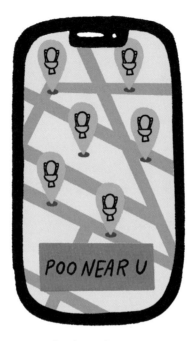

**Technology: Getting you
where you want to go.**

near me" in the search bar and usually get decent results. Google Maps allows users to save specific geolocations to a list, so as you encounter more public toilets in your area, they can be saved to the toilet archives. You can also easily share these lists with others, so some major cities like New York have a map online of all the free public toilets that you can download to your device.

GAS IN THE TANK

Once a few toilet options are known, you now gotta look deep inside yourself and determine your fuel level.[9] If you're running on empty, then great, you can go the extra mile to get that clean and safe restroom. However, if you've got a tank (colon) full of gas (actually just gas), you might want to over-index on proximity. Knowing your body in these situations is critical.

TIME TO DECIDE

Now you can make the most informed decision about where to spend your toilet time. But are you willing to pay for your experience? More and more establishments are taking a "Customers Only" bathroom policy to stop good, hardworking folks like yourself from finding restroom relief. This book thinks you can do better, so don't panic and buy a stale croissant—take up the challenge and get the bathroom code for free. Agent 002 is here to help.

---

9   Your body has an inverse relationship with gas as compared to a car, in terms of toilet needs—running on empty is ideal.

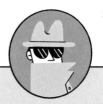

AGENT 002 MISSION

Oh, the Places You'll Go!

Your next mission: Find a free toilet to use in public, on the double! Use your peripheral vision to scan your surroundings, and keep these tips in mind as you make your meticulous moves:

1. Big, crowded establishments are your best friend here. **Find the nearest nice hotel with a lobby**—but not too nice, because the door person and bellhops will try to talk to you, and for all you know they may know every guest by sight. I've had the best luck with mid-tier giant hotel chains. Do not try a motel; they usually have no lobby bathroom, and I don't recommend knocking on room doors. If someone asks what room you're staying in, act like you didn't hear them. If that doesn't work, #402 is usually a safe answer, assuming the hotel has that many floors.[10]

2. If you go the fast-food route, at least pick a place with food you enjoy; that way you can have a guilty pleasure afterward as a treat.[11]

---

10 Hotels really are your best friend here; the lobby bathrooms are nice and pretty private! I even use the lobby restroom when I'm a guest at the hotel to keep my room smelling fresh.

11 Let's be honest: Fast food tastes amazing.

3. Public transportation hubs, malls, department stores, and libraries usually have free restroom options, and no awkward interaction is needed for the restroom key/pin. But in the case that it is, at least you're in a high-traffic area, so you can quickly dissolve into the crowd.
4. Gas stations and outdoor kiosks are always hit or miss. Usually free (with a key/pin code), but the real danger here is the state of cleanliness.
5. Often surprisingly difficult: coffee shops or pharmacy store chains. They take their public bathroom protection seriously, for some reason.

No matter what, stay cool and confident, act casual, and do your best to blend in. And remember, I will always be with you if you get in a bind.[12] Good luck!

SECURITY

True story time: Once as a young boy I was using my bathroom at home. I did not lock the door, and my Great Grandma (with dementia) busted in and pulled me off the toilet because she had to go. I'm assuming it was an emergency. Not only do I remain confused about that whole situation, but to this day I now remember my GG in that

12   Well, that is, if you carry this book with you everywhere.

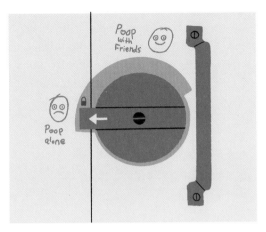

You decide.

weird way. But I was like four—it's understandable that I forgot to lock the door. I'm guessing you are not four, so LOCK THE DOOR.

You are embarking on one of life's most vulnerable situations; don't accidentally share this hot and heavy moment with others like I did. For the stall-door slide-lock hooks, make sure they are wedged all the way and the door is secured.[13] Take the extra time to test with a few quick pulls before taking a seat.

After securing the door, you also MUST do a quick check that there's enough toilet paper available to get the job done. More to come on this later, but it's equally as important as securing the situation.

13 This "pretend shut" situation is a sneaky surprise for amateurs. Especially on rusty door locks that could use some WD-40.

KNOCKING ON THE BATHROOM DOOR

Why do people knock on the door when the restroom is locked? It's clearly occupied by someone having a private moment who is almost certainly uninterested in communication. Just don't do it. Also, people having to wait for anything just generally brings out the worst in humanity.

YOUR PORT IN THE STORM: STALL SELECTION

When entering these public bathrooms, you're faced with the unique but ultimate decision: Which one do I pick? Make the wrong choice and you'll be working your quads, hovering over the seat, holding your breath—whereas making the right choice lets you spread out and enjoy a brief moment of tranquility. So let's dive deeper into the strategy of stall selection.

Hello and welcome to *Let's Find A Stall*, a game played every time we enter a public bathroom, where our toilet fate lies behind three mysterious stall-type-door options. Are you ready to begin? Now I will do the thing where I tell you about each option to build tension on the decision!

STALL DOOR #1: THE FIRST STALL (CLOSEST TO THE DOOR)

Coming in as the first option is the first edge stall! Behind this door you'll be rewarded with just one stall neighbor and the scent of fresh air because you're closest to the door! But your next-door neighbor is the sink area, so your feet have the highest probability of sitting in puddles because you are certainly in the splash zone. However, MythBusters discovered this stall is typically the least used, which means less bacteria exposure for you behind this door!

STALL DOOR #2: THE MIDDLE STALL

Just like the middle seat on an airplane, this door is rarely chosen, even though it will still get you to your destination. This stall is usually available and can be a solid choice if the neighboring stalls are also empty. Butttttt you might also find yourself absorbing all the sounds and smells of your neighbors because you're stuck in a super stall sandwich.[14]

STALL DOOR #3: THE CORNER STALL (FARTHEST FROM THE DOOR)

And finally, behind our final door option is the corner stall, the penthouse suite of public restrooms. This unit typically has the most amount of privacy because it's

---

14 Not the five-dollar footlong sub you might be hoping for.

the farthest from the door and sometimes only has a
stall neighbor on one side and some extra legroom.
Baby changing stations are commonly found in these
if that benefit means anything to you.

(ASK PLUNGIE)

Silent Stall Standoff

Sometimes schedules align such that you and a
stall neighbor's bowel movements end up perfectly
in sync. For the shy among us, this risks entering
into a classic silent stall standoff, where both of you
quietly wait for the other person to finish before
you start going. This results in both parties, well,
stalling in each stall. Break the silence barrier with
these decoy sounds, which should free you up to go
about your business:

- **Toilet Roll Holder:** Getting toilet paper makes
  so much noise and indicates to the other party
  that you are further along in the process,
  hopefully prompting them to make noise.
- **Cough:** One or two coughs, short and sharp.
- **Sneezing:** This involves a bit more of a
  performance, but it's also kind of fun.
- **Just Go for It:** As long as you don't
  exit at the same time as them, you'll
  always just be anonymous anyways.

STALL GRAFFITI APPRECIATION

The German artist Joseph Beuys once said, "Everyone is an artist," and it goes without saying that everyone uses the toilet. Ergo, the potential to discover art on stall walls is high, and every stall has a story to share. Most works will be of the Figurative (Stick) variety, and indeed, the stall arts also tend more to the literary. Generally unsigned, these anonymous works of wit may be colored in a spectrum of hues from confession to accusation, outrage to admiration, self-promotion, manifesto, exclamation, testimonials, jokes, denunciations, and beyond. Like all art, stall graffiti comes from the ideas of the individuals who create it, in this case the restroom community. And while Andy Warhol's axiom of everyone being "world famous" for fifteen minutes may not fulfill its global reach here, within the stall an artist's fame may extend far into future bathroom visitations (depending on how often the walls are repainted).

Remember, no two stalls are the same—always inspect before you commit to sit. Find a lurker in the bowl? Pay it forward by flushing it down and checking the next stall. Nasty puddles? Dry land may be found next door. Mission critical: *Is there enough toilet paper?*

28

⇨ **RANDOM SHORT RANT** ☺
SAY NO TO CRACKS!

Why are there cracks or open gaps in bathroom stall
walls? It doesn't have to be this way. WE HAVE THE
TECHNOLOGY to seal these sanctuaries and end
awkward mind-the-gap eye contact once and for all!
Maximum Acceptable Stall Crack Width: 0 inches!

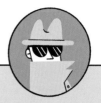

`AGENT 002 MISSION`

Shoes under Stalls

Your mission is to collect as much information on
your neighboring stall suspects WITHOUT engaging
them. In this game, every character that crosses
paths with you has a history, and it's up to you to
make it up for them. Scan for details on their footwear, for example:

- **Fancy dress shoes:** just got married
  or interviewing for job
- **Fancy dress shoes + crying:** wedding or
  interview didn't go well

- **Sandals:** folk singer, beach bum, or both
- **Crocs:** they either worked an 8-hour counter shift, or have given up on life, or are fashion forward (Crocs are back, baby)
- **Skates, skateboard, or Heelys:** probably Tony Hawk

Try it out yourself. Sneakers, boots, flip-flops: Each one tells a story. Best believe we have double agents keeping tabs on your shoes too. Always show off your freshest footwear in the bathroom so you can win at this guessing game.

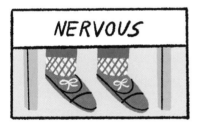

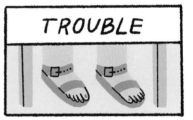

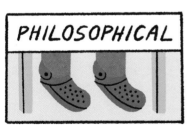

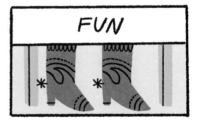

Who are you?

A GRACEFUL EXIT (THE SINK SITUATION)

You have just emerged from a glorious experience (hopefully), and now you're semi-back in society, but nobody knows exactly how to interact with each other. Do we avoid eye contact? Do we acknowledge each other? What if I just used the last piece of paper towel and people are waiting behind me?

Here are some recommended do's and don'ts for navigating the fraught terrain separating you from rejoining the outside world.

- **Grant Space:** Don't be that person who hovers behind someone while they are using the sink. Back up, give folks some elbow room to scrub, and wait your turn.[15]

- **Scope the Sink:** Do look down before getting close to the sink to see if the countertops are soaked. You don't want to brush up against that while rinsing and then get those awkward wet stains right above your crotch.[16] Sink runoff spills all over the floor and really can make this area slippery, so be careful and keep your kicks looking spiffy.

- **Speaking of Slipping:** If things have become bad enough for someone to place one of those signs

---

15 People also do this at airport baggage claim, and it makes the process of getting your bag so much harder.
16 Something I always stress about when using the bathroom right before an interview.

depicting a figure who looks either like they're ska dancing or waving to you from the spot they found on the beach, do trust that things are as swampy as advertised and watch your step.

- **Points for Cleanliness:** If you're going to shoot hoops with your paper towel and the trash receptacle, either be infallible or be willing to pick it up and dunk it yourself.
- **Think before You Drink:** Are you literally dying of thirst? If not, don't drink directly from the sink tap, you unsanitary monster. It looks gross, it sounds gross, and it contributes to wet floors and countertops (see second bullet).

CROSSING PATHS

Sometimes when exiting a mission, you'll perfectly cross paths with another person that goes straight into the stall or bathroom you just left.[17] If it was a messy venture, you have an opportunity to be a Good Samaritan and warn them of any land mines you might have uncovered or caused (i.e., you just used the last piece of toilet paper). Always leave the state of the situation better than when you found it, looking out for the next person (more on

---

17 This is very illogical, but every time this happens to me, it always feels like an invasion of privacy. Like dude, give it a second, you know? Toilets should always have an idle barrier of time between customers.

the Leave No Trace philosophy later). At some point we realize that we're all going to be the next person too.

ROBOTS RUINING RESTROOMS

Automation is coming for our jobs, even in the bathroom. And they're bad at it!

- **Sinks:** The hand sensor is difficult to trigger, flow time is never long enough, and the pressure is meh. I wanna get all the soap suds off my hands up to MY standard before the all-knowing sink cuts off.

- **Flushers:** These toilets are way too trigger-happy. Don't even get me started on this one. Life hack: Cover the little sensor with a piece of toilet paper, and it won't flush until you take it off. You'll take back control from the robots.[18]

- **Dryers:** Not only do these blowers leave your hands drippy, but they also spread fecal aerosols all over your hands and the restroom. The *MythBusters* folks ran a test and found that hand dryers created ten times the bacteria colonies around the bathroom after being used.

---

18 Also, if you've ever thought your life was a simulation, don't watch one of these toilets get stuck in a flush loop. It's a mesmerizing but scary cycle.

Fast & Furious Flushing

One of the biggest positives for pooping in public is that you are most likely sitting on a *commercial* toilet (*industrial grade*), the silverback gorillas of the toilet kingdom. But what makes a toilet fit into this category? Well, commercial toilets do not have a holding tank connected on the back and instead flush directly from a water line, which has more pressure. A home toilet connects to a floating tank and valve, which has a lower flush capacity but also uses less water.

Many folks are now considering a commercial toilet in their home because it takes up less space (no holding tank) and is much harder to clog. But most residential water piping lacks enough flow and pressure to support a toilet without a tank.

However, there is a dark side to these super flushers! Sometimes their jet power is so strong that it creates hot tub–like movement in the bowl, which can cause major sprinkler-effect splash back. I *especially* recommend flushing these with the toilet lid (and your mouth) closed.

SO IT'S COME TO THIS: PORTA-POTTIES

Every video game has a final boss, and you have just been introduced to the biggest challenge while out in public—The Porta-Potty. For whatever reason (the plastic construction, the outdoor location external to society's norms, or the long lines and desperation customers feel when arriving), people seem to behave especially unhygienically in these desperate crap shacks, and you may be in for a unique sensory experience. If you find yourself facing this particular challenge, ask yourself: Is this truly my best or only option?

The strategy here is to get in, get out, and get away from said porta-potty as quickly as you can. Be thankful that there is a bathroom for you at this moment of need, but also be mad that you didn't plan ahead better. DO NOT TOUCH the sketchy blue liquid,[19] and be sure to keep your wiping form shallow. Since there's a non-zero percent chance the toilet paper will give you a rash, consider carrying large tissues and hand sanitizer with you at all times (see p. 38, To-Go Bags). Upon your exit, especially if you are in an area you frequent or may return to, take a minute to consider other options that could be better toilets for next time. Your future self will thank you!

---

19   It's not blue Gatorade, which happens to be the best flavor.

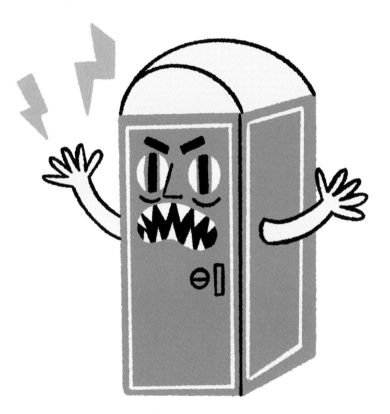

Challenge accepted.

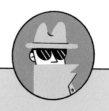

AGENT 002 MISSION

Touch Nothing

We need you to get in that porta-potty, get the job
done, and get out WITHOUT making hand contact
with any surface. Do not ask me why. It's too gross
to explain. Ultimately, you will have to be creative to
accomplish this mission, but here are some ideas to
get you started:

- If the porta-potty is occupied previous to your
  turn, try to catch the door with your back or
  butt as the other person leaves. This avoids
  you having to grab the handle.
- Wrap your hands in toilet paper like a boxing
  glove. A very thin layer is still a layer, and
  you need to be prepared to go ten rounds in
  this ring.
- Hover over the seat when dropping the
  package.
- Use your elbows when necessary to push open
  the door or keep it open when entering.
- Not really related to surface contact, but just
  hold your breath for your own happiness.
  For especially odiferous situations, consider
  toilet paper nose plugs.

STAYING SANITARY

One of the biggest worries when using a public toilet is the unknown exposure to germs. While every public toilet is unique in terms of cleanliness, studies of infectious disease transmission identified the biggest risk areas when using the facilities.

- **Toilet Bowl:** No surprises here, this contains the most bacteria and viruses due to feces and urine. Flushing with the seat cover down helps contain these microbes from entering the air you breathe. They can reach five feet in the air and sit there for an hour after just one flush.

- **Toilet Seat:** Again not a huge surprise, but luckily most infections aren't butt-borne, so you should be okay. Flushable seat covers can help, as can a strategic placement of toilet paper strips in lieu of a seat cover, but disinfectant spray is the best way to eliminate bacteria before sitting. Or hover, if you can!

- **Bathroom Floor:** Hey guess what? The floor hosts many germs too. Try hanging your jacket, bag, or purse on a door hook instead of putting it on the ground.

- **Phone:** A favorite of many folks' toilet time, but sadly, keeping this in your pocket is the best way for you to avoid germs getting on your phone, which means all over your hands.

TO-GO BAGS

A field agent is only as good as their gadgets, so now's your chance to pack your equipment bag when out and about on missions. Purses are pretty big these days, and most of these items can also be easily stored in a back-pack or fanny pack (they're back in style!) or car side door. Here are my favorites:

- **Toilet Tissue To-Go:** Never worry about wiping again—these can easily fit in a pocket.
- **Toilet Seat Sanitizer Spray:** Nobody likes sitting on those crinkly paper wraps—go ahead and cancel all your future butt dermatologist appointments.
- **Hand Sanitizer:** A great way to sterilize them wipers if the sink situation isn't ideal, or if you are in a porta-potty.
- **Wet Wipe:** These can be used on the toilet seat or your human seat.

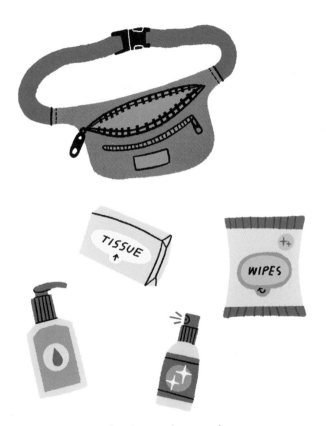

The ultimate fanny pack.

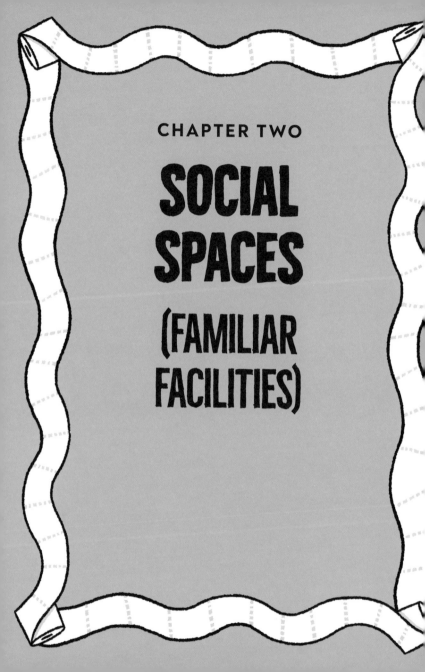

CHAPTER TWO

SOCIAL SPACES

(FAMILIAR FACILITIES)

WORK AND SCHOOL

A lucky few may never step foot into an office again, but most of us will continue commuting to our "contribution to society," which means we must navigate the restroom while on the clock. To many the idea of going during work or school can be something we dread, a too-intimate form of digestive oversharing. But going among professional peers is all about knowing how to play the game, and it's time to get your butt promoted.[20]

WHY YOU SHOULD

PAID TO POOP

Do you live in a capitalistic society? Hey, me too! What could be more on-brand than monetizing your bowel schedule? Accumulate some passive income while you are on the toilet. Naturally, this also means you should be holding in all your poo on the weekends and waiting until Monday to release, when you are back on the clock (obviously kidding).

---

20 Ideally, your butt never has to report to another butt ever again.

TAKE TIME

The end-of-day clock countdown doesn't stop even if
you do! Take as much time as you need on the throne,
returning to your desk knowing you are closer to evening
freedom. Work smarter, not harder.

BUDGETING

Becoming an adult[21] has shown me that stocking your
bathroom at home is weirdly kind of expensive. The average consumer spends roughly $20 a month on bathroom
essentials. Make your company or local school pay for
your supplies to poop!

HOLDING IT IN IS A SIN!

Holding in your poop (literal toxins) is not good for you
and can have annoying health side effects like constipation, impaction, hemorrhoids, and sometimes even inflam-
mation of the colon. Work/school days are a minimum of
eight hours in length, which is way too long to be stress-
fully holding in a storm.

GREAT ESCAPES: WORK/SCHOOL EDITION

A key trick to surviving the rest of your professional/
educational life: Go to the bathroom even when you don't
have to "go." Not feeling sentence-structure grammar

rules at 9 a.m.? Go to the bathroom! Hungover, or feel like every decision is just too much? Go to the bathroom! Your rival coworker just took credit for something you did in the team sync? Go to the bathroom! Your crush checked NO to your prom invite? Go to the bathroom in a different school!

You get the point: Going to the bathroom solves— or at least postpones—almost every temporary problem. Everyone at some point needs a *Mean Girls*–style solo lunch in a bathroom stall.

ASK PLUNGIE
Calendar Craziness

Is your workday stacked with meeting after meeting? Do you frequently get asked to "sit in" or "weigh in" on meetings that really don't concern you? Everyone should have time to use the bathroom, so take back your calendar! If you find yourself overscheduled, block off don't-bother-me windows of time for bathroom breaks. Most calendar systems have a handy private meeting feature that just shows you as busy; but if it doesn't, here are a few ideas for what to fill in for the calendar blocks:

- **"Quick Sync"**: This classic is never questioned; communication is key! "Touch Base" is also a solid option here too.

- **"Brainstorm":** People love a good word cloud in corporate environments.
- **"Strategy Session":** Bonus points if you happen to be a consultant.
- **"Debrief Dump":** Sharing is caring.
- **"Bathroom Break":** Just own it; everybody's gotta go.
- **"NONE OF YOUR BUSINESS":** Your calendar, your life.

HAVE A PLAN

One of the easiest things about using the toilet in these settings is that nothing about the setup should be uncertain, unless of course it's your first day. You've had plenty of time to study the game tape and develop a playbook, so you should be quite familiar with your options. Here are additional considerations I've used for professionally pooping:

- **Backup Bathroom:** Always have one in case your main squeeze is having a moment. Kudos if they are on different floors to really create separation in schedules.
- **Know Your Calendar:** Each day can be different; own your schedule! If you have a big presentation coming up, make sure to get your toilet time in before.

- **Heat Map:** Where do bodies congregate typically in the building? Any abandoned wings or floors that don't see a lot of foot traffic? When do your coworkers come and go?[22]
- **My Homies:** When do your closest peers (classmates, teammates, managers) go? These observations may feel creepy, but they prevent some awkward situations.
- **Company All-Hands Meetings and School Announcements:** The perfect opportunity to avoid brainwashing and get the best bathroom in the building, so look out for these calendar invites.
- **Kicks:** Don't wear flashy shoes or call attention to your sneakers, because people will remember them and then be able to identify you under stall doors.
- **Swapping Shoes:** If you see yourself as a sneaker-head, or if you just have a signature staple shoe, odds are that your coworkers and classmates have noticed (or maybe even admired) your footwear. Consider swapping out your nice kicks for poo shoes to remain anonymous in shared stall spaces, and also to keep your everyday cleats clean.

22 This is real life, not the beginning of a horror film, so this should be pretty safe. Unless you start to see flickering lights . . .

HOME AWAY FROM HOME

Research has shown that those who travel for work get better sleep if they stay consistently at the same hotel, because they are in a familiar environment where they feel safe. Most people poop every day. Enhance your own sense of comfort, and help avoid pooping in scary new places, by having some go-to options when on the go. Pre-scouted facilities at work and school—where you spend roughly 33 percent of your life[23]—can offer you this sort of oasis.

WHEN TO AVOID

RUSH HOUR

The bathroom, where we want to be alone and anonymous, isn't a safe space if all your coworkers are there too. Do you really want to know what Jerry from Accounting's bottom burps sound like? Here are times to avoid an awkward hand-washing conversation at the sink:

- **9:30 to 10:30 a.m.:** Everyone has just arrived and are fighting depression through the consumption of coffee. Soon they will need to flush out these feelings, so try to squeeze your morning poop in early or right before lunch.

---

23 This statistic is a little depressing, but yeah, you're gonna be going a lot at work throughout your life.

- **1:00 to 2:30 p.m.:** Ah, the post-lunch-partum poop, where you are at the will of whatever was served in the cafeteria, from food trucks, or as noontime specials that day. Especially avoid this time if your office had catering for lunch brought in—it's usually something greasy, and everyone feasted at the same time, so they are on the same digestive schedule. Nothing quite beats up a bathroom like former attendees of a pizza party.

If you must absolutely go during these times, try a different floor of the office or wing of the school. Less risk for crossing paths with a familiar face.

Plan ahead to avoid high-traffic times. Consider taking a load off before you leave for the day.

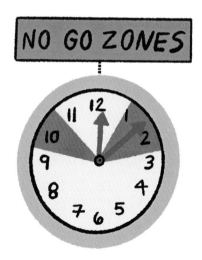

FIRE DRILLS

This is a toss-up—on one hand you are pretty much guaranteed an empty bathroom all to yourself. On the other hand, if you're in too long, you'll be missed in the safety headcount outside. You might also be wrong about it being a "drill."

LAYOFFS/PERFORMANCE REVIEWS

People will likely be in the stalls crying, which will make your soiling time sad, and also not private. Especially perilous when the economy is in a recession.

VALENTINE'S DAY/PROM NIGHT

Same as above—broken hearts, or potentially even worse, *horny hearts*, will be using the stall space.

RIVALS ROAMING

Everybody has an adversary in their life. They might just be uniquely annoying, or worse, an actual enemy: the school bully or Tina from Marketing with her Machiavellian scheming. Don't give them an unsupervised opportunity with you; make sure their desk is occupied before you head out to do your thing.

⇨ **RANDOM SHORT RANT** ☺
BATHROOM BANTER

We've all been in a casual conversation with someone that quickly became not chill when you both realized that you were heading toward the bathroom. But to make it worse, neither of you knew how to end it as you both continued into adjacent stalls. *Just don't do this.* Conversations should cease when a bathroom is entered, to preserve the safe zone. But more importantly, just avoid rush hour altogether to decrease the likelihood of this happening.

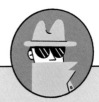

`AGENT 002 MISSION`
Water Closet Whispers

Not everyone adheres to the safe zone belief, so the restroom sanctum is sometimes ruined with chatter. In these circumstances enter the area with your eyes and ears open, as intelligence is floating everywhere. Want to hear the latest gossip about why somebody didn't get the promotion? The bathroom.

Want to buy some rare Pokémon cards from Jimmy
in fifth period? The bathroom. No notes need to be
passed, bullies can freely flex their fists, and your
director won't be in there, because they have their
own private bath connected to their corner office.
Find out the real 411 when things in the real world
seem suspiciously fun.

OTHER PEOPLE'S HOUSES

The stakes are high here for two reasons: 1) you probably have
a relationship with the toilet owner that you would like to keep,
and 2) they likely don't have a commercial toilet that is being
cleaned and maintained by a paid professional. That means
that your toilet experience will be shaped by existing circumstances (just like any time you are going away from home),
but also now you have an extra social obligation to navigate in
terms of demonstrating good bathroom citizenship. Don't let
your behind betray your besties—this is the time to perform
the skill of discreetly defecating.

FAR AND AWAY: FINDING THE BEST OPTION

Bathroom location within a private domain is still everything. Do you really wanna be blowing up the half bath connected to the kitchen while the rest of the fam is making Christmas cookies? Only amateurs use bathrooms closest to the action. The key ingredient here is the toilet's relative distance to the social situation.

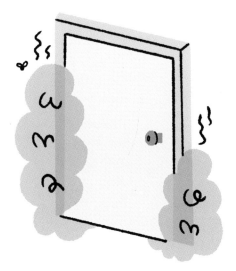

**Find a bathroom as far as possible from
where folks are gathered.**

Whenever you enter a new private domain, ask the host for a home tour[24] or just go on a self-guided tour. Aside from admiring the homeowner's creepy porcelain doll collection, also take note of the various porcelain throne bathroom options, keeping the following in mind:

- The "master bathroom" is likely to be the most cushy and well-stocked. It's also kind of an inner sanctum space, which might be awkward ("Oh, hi, Brad. Didn't expect to find you back here . . ."). But it's also going to be your most satisfying option in terms of snooping opportunities. What brand of toilet paper do they have? Does it seem like they're flossing? How's their skincare routine?

- The most remote option, in the garage/basement/sub-basement/bomb shelter, is going to give you the most privacy, but it's also more likely to be neglected in terms of upkeep and TP stock.[25] Also, folks who venture to these quiet corners tend to get murdered first in every Hollywood horror movie.

- A good rule of thumb: One floor above or below the main action is likely to be your best bet for an undisturbed (and undisturbing for others) experience.

---

24 This is a win-win: You get the information you need, and they get the validation of talking about their decorative choices.

25 Actually, the bomb shelter is probably well stocked. A safe place to drop a bomb of your own?

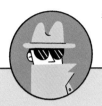

AGENT 002 MISSION

Homemade Door Lock

Think quick, the only bathroom available has no door lock! In this mission, you must battle architectural constraints[26] and find a way to secure the perimeter. Look to see if there's a sink cabinet or drawer near the door and pull it out to create a makeshift barrier. If not, look for another item in the bathroom that could be used to wedge the door instead. You might have to use your foot!

AMENITIES

These remote outposts aren't being supervised and restocked with supplies when they get low. This is why you do recon! Make sure the bathroom has all the essentials that you need for success. Then see how many bonus amenities you got as well. Before you squat, save yourself from some stress.

- **Essentials:** toilet, toilet paper, sink, soap, plunger
- **Bonus:** backup toilet paper, fan, window, reading materials, modern art, deodorizing products, shower/tub (worst-case), breath mints

Make absolutely sure your chosen spot has all of the essentials (TOILET PAPER) before shutting the door to do your business. Do not assume that your friends always have this in stock, especially in guest bathrooms.

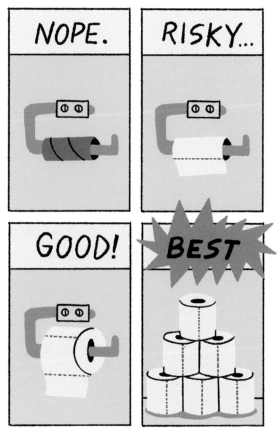

Choose wisely.

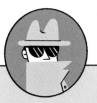

AGENT 002 MISSION

Supplies Shortage

This next challenge might be the toughest you'll face yet—realizing you are almost out of toilet paper during the middle of a squat session. As an elite agent, you've been trained not to panic. You've got this.

- If you have some left, ration the rest up to the last teeny tiny bit. Wipe conservatively and strategically, no unnecessary nose blowing.
- Double-check for backup TP behind the toilet or under the sink. Make note if you find paper towels or facial tissues.
- When all the toilet paper runs out, you can:
  » Use a very small amount of paper towels/tissues to complete the job; just don't clog their toilet or damage their piping.
  » The center cardboard roll actually works quite well if you break up into pieces.[27] Wet it under the sink to increase softness before scraping.

NEVER ASSUME SOMEONE HAS AN ADEQUATE AMOUNT OF TP.

27 People wipe with sticks in the wild. I promise a little cardboard won't hurt you!

PORCELAIN PROTOCOL

As good bathroom citizens, we must always strive to Leave No Trace (when you leave the bathroom, it should look like you were never there), especially when we're guests in someone else's home. Some considerations:

SOUNDS

Everyone's butt can be a little loud sometimes, and there's no shame in that. But for the sake of all your friends listening to your water closet concert, try to create as much white noise to cover your "brown noise" as possible.

- If there's a fan, turn it on. It'll help with any odor as well as add cover sound.
- Run the sink. Not full-taps open, but the sound of freshwater flow can help.
- Play music. Make it a concert of actual noncolonic music.
- Sing. No music? Sing from your above to cover singing from your below.
- Run bath/shower. For extreme circumstances, it's like the sink times one thousand for white noise. You might get some questions. Saying I wanted to rinse my feet mostly works for me.

SMELLS

Unfortunately, we all know people that loudly pro-
claim whoever left the bathroom smelly. And it's
understandable: A terrible scent leaving a toilet can
ruin any board game night. Don't just reactively say
sorry.[28] Some of these may seem obvious, but employ-
ing them ahead of the squat may help you avoid some
smelly situations.

- Again, turn on the fan.
- Crack open a window.
- Deploy in-process courtesy flush(es) to get the waste
  down the tubes ASAP.
- Find air fresheners or matches[29] for afterward.
- Keep the window open and fan running when leaving.
- [OPTIONAL] Open and close the toilet seat rapidly
  to get air moving, like a manual fan.
- Close the bathroom door behind you (DUH).

28 Unless you're playing Sorry at board game night.
29 Maybe you're like me and don't like air fresheners. But if you've found them in someone
    else's bathroom, it means they do. Use 'em. And the match trick still blows my mind—
    that's my favorite.

58

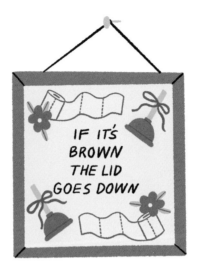

Words to live by.

ASK PLUNGIE

Lower the Lid

We already mentioned that flushing your feces with the lid open allows bacteria particles to enter the air, but it also frees smelly odor droplets to escape into the air! What we smell is directly due to physical interactions, so putting the toilet seat down when flushing the mess keeps you healthier and a bathroom smelling fresher, which is a cause your friend's house can get behind.

TRACE EVIDENCE

So your bowels have taken this inopportune time to leave an abstract expressionist masterpiece of digestive artwork on the bowl that is now somehow unmoved by flushing (toilet bowl stains). Don't panic and just keep at it: Sometimes the third flush is the charm. If the tire tracks are really there to stay, a quick swipe with a toilet scrubber or plunger can help manage the damage. Without those tools at hand, it's time to make yourself a TP glove, hit flush, and swipe the problem area in the brief window when the bowl is basically empty before refilling. Flush the "glove" and wash your hands. However, like most creative pursuits, interpretation for cleaning skid marks is up to said artist.[30] For those who despise scrubbing the toilet bowl, there are automatic cleaners you can install that get the job done quite well and leave a refreshing scent for next time!

FLUSHING FAILS: A RISK ASSESSMENT

The number one goal when going number two at a friend's pad should be avoiding a clogged toilet. The stress of seeing the water rise, desperately shutting off the toilet's water tap before overflow, and then having to ask for a plunger can ruin any chill hang. So be one step ahead, and don't clog the toilet by staying under the *flush capacity* (the breaking-point volume a toilet can handle in a single flush).

How can you tell the threshold of a toilet you've never used? Here are some tips so that you can flush with confidence:

- Check flush capacity. Sometimes this is printed directly on the toilet: 1.0 GPF (gallons per flush) and below is low, 1.28 GPF is the new water-saving standard, and 1.6 GPF or more is high.

- Single vs dual flush: You definitely want to use the dual button when given this option.

- Is the seat small or the toilet height short? These are signs you are sitting on an older toilet model, so be extra careful about clogging. They may have a higher flush volume (pre-efficiency laws), but they may also have narrower drainpipes, less powerful flush valves, and had more time to accrue mineral buildup that lowers the water pressure even more.

- The presence of flushable wipes in someone's bathroom indicates a more powerful toilet.

- BEWARE of the slow flushers (low pressure) where the turd rides around the bowl like a lazy river. If it keeps circling on numerous flushes, throw a wet blanket of TP over its little party and let physics help speed it down.

- AND WATCH OUT for handles with lots of give. Hold those unsteady suckers down longer to keep the flow going.

FLUSH FREQUENTLY

If you have any doubts about the clogging risk you may face, employ the courtesy flush, early and often, so material doesn't accumulate, and before TP is even a factor. You're giving the toilet manageable milestones instead of a big, scary problem (like any manager should). This tactic is a bit water wasteful, but in this moment avoiding a clog should be the priority. Be sure to briefly pause a few moments between flushes, so the toilet can refill and recharge.

CLOGGING THE TOILET

The words your host least wants to hear from you are "It's clogged." Be the hero in this moment and clean up your bathroom big bang, or at least try and manage the damage. Though if you don't know the owner and have a 50/50 chance you might never see them again, leaving through the window isn't a bad plan either.

If you followed my earlier advice and picked a bathroom with a plunger, you might just be able to erase this situation without public attention. Run the sink to create some white noise, roll up your sleeves, and get to it. Clear the floor area of any bath mats before taking the plunge, because you are in the splash zone. When finished, rinse the plunger in the bowl's fresh toilet water[31] and place the plunger in the wastebasket or find a trash bag to contain the toxins. Give the host a heads-up there's a hot plunger in the house.[32] If they don't own a plunger . . . they don't own a plunger?

EMERGING BACK INTO SOCIETY

It's time to rejoin the world a little lighter! Unfortunately, out of sight does not always mean out of mind, and if your mission was lengthy, your reappearance might draw some attention. An easy way to explain the length of your absence is to pair the toilet time with an additional task. Peek into a room near the restroom, grab a book or tchotchke off a shelf, and walk in asking a question about it. Or walk in holding your phone up to your face and pretend to be wrapping up a phone call ("I love you too, Mom, call you later!"). If attention is unavoidable, or maybe attention is your thing, own it and offer a "you do NOT want to go in there" to acknowledge and move on.

---

31 As a bonus, look for disinfectant spray under the sink while you are rinsing the plunger.

32 If you can't find a plunger but can find a toilet bowl brush (for some reason?), a Hail Mary strategy could be to chop up the blockage into smaller pieces with the brush and see if they flush down. The brush cleanup is pretty similar to the plunger, so it's really not a bad escape option.

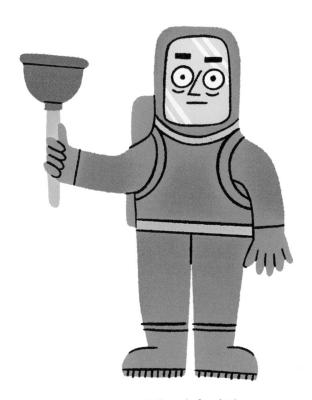

Y'all ready for this?

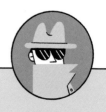

AGENT 002 MISSION

The Stealth Shower

You find yourself in a difficult situation—you've been at it for twenty-plus minutes (red zone for toilet time) and have completed the mission, but now you are sweaty and no longer in social shape to hang. You need to explain your absence and come back to the party smelling fresh—you need to take a *Stealth Shower.* Planning your poops with other bathroom activities like shaving, showering, and brushing your teeth can buy ten to fifteen more minutes of explicable bathroom time, certainly if you're in your own home. At someone else's place, read vibes and who's present to determine if an impromptu shower would be actually transgressive.

GREAT ESCAPES: SOCIAL EDITION

We talked about escaping from your professional respon-
sibilities on the toilet, but this strategy also works just as
well for your social life. Maybe your ex just walked into the
party? Or your nosy relative won't stop asking when you
and your partner are going to have kids. Once you're done
with the task at hand, give yourself a minute. Freshen up,
make sure everything looks solid in the mirror, and give
yourself a pep talk, or a quiet moment of Zen, before your
reemergence.

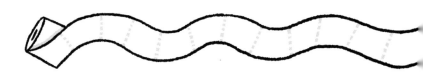

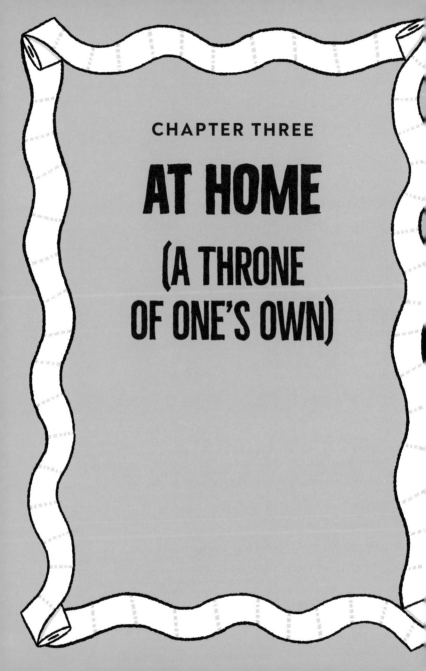

CHAPTER THREE

AT HOME
(A THRONE OF ONE'S OWN)

HOME SWEET HOME

It's time focus on the personal privy palace, your one toilet to rule them all and your butt's best friend: THE HOME TOILET.

According to Nick Haslam, professor of psychology and author of *Psychology in the Bathroom*, there's a biological reason why we have a sigh of relief when entering our home after a long day or trip away. When in an unfamiliar environment, our sensory receptors are constantly updating us about new inputs and considerations, which causes our adrenaline to be higher and more fat deposits to be burned. It even impacts our rate of digestion and food moving through our stomach. So when returning home, our sensory stimulation is lower and our relaxation response kicks in, making it easier and generally much more pleasant to poop.

But on a different wavelength, there have been quite a few famous fatalities on home toilets. In some ways it makes sense; we spend so much time there folks are bound to be on one in their final moments. But the track record is shocking: many members of the historic royal family, Elvis Presley, Judy Garland, and even Coolio.[33]

33 This has inspired many throne deaths in film and media: *Jurassic Park*, *Game of Thrones*, *Pulp Fiction*, *South Park*, *Saturday Night Live*, *Succession* . . .

TRICKING OUT THE THRONE ROOM, PART ONE: PORCELAIN PRACTICALITY

Using the bathroom at home should be easy, even pleasurable. It's often said that investing in your bed is really an investment in yourself due to the increased sleep quality. Well, the toilet is no different. These battles take place in your arena, which means you should have full home-court advantage. But how does one create the perfect poop environment? It's time to trick out the throne room!

ON A ROLL

The average person uses eighty-five rolls of toilet paper each year, and our IBS readers, including me, can go many more than that. This adds up to almost four hundred trees of toilet paper—a little forest!—in one's lifetime![34] Sure, when out and about, one must deal with the paper provided. But at home, this is your chance to optimize what matters most to you—your pocketbook, your bum, or the planet.

---

34 Twenty-seven thousand trees are used worldwide each day, translating to ten million every year. TP is the printed currency of the bathroom economy, and the third-largest polluting industry.

HOW IT'S MADE: TERMS OF MATERIALS

Standard

Unless otherwise stated, you can assume any white toilet paper you are using is chlorine bleached. These chemicals are found on most of our printed paper products and do enter our body and bloodstream as dioxins. But there are alternatives, usually labeled as "Chlorine Free" and "Unbleached," that avoid the chemical processes. Bleaching doesn't just turn it white; it also makes the paper softer to the touch. Therefore, natural variations are usually a bit rougher.

Recycled (Pre- and Post-Consumer)

Naturally, one might think this is toilet paper reincarnated for a second session, but it's actually just generally recycled paper materials—newspapers, magazines, books, etc. This paper can be post- (already used by people) or pre- (leftover materials never used) consumer, so this option is better for the environment, as it uses half the water and creates a third of the greenhouse gases compared to virgin pulp paper processes. Recycled *can* still contain chemical compounds such as BPA (given the original paper had it) and unfortunately is also not known to be the softest.

Bamboo

Standard TP is sourced from wood pulp, which contributes massively to our paper deforestation. This kind
comes from bamboo trees (surprise, surprise), which grow
twenty times faster than trees in northern forests, and the
paper-making process emits *30 percent* fewer greenhouse
gases. It doesn't have quite the environmental savings of
recycled toilet paper, but it's generally more comfortable,
so it's the best of both worlds.

Single-Ply

This single layer of paper is typically found in most public
restrooms—it's cost effective but rough. Even though it
tears easily, it's very low-flush friendly for sensitive septic
tanks and is often found in boats and RVs for that reason.

Multi-Ply

Multiple-ply (two, three, and even four) are just single-
paper plies glued together to make a more durable
square. More plies come with additional wiping protection, but also more density that your piping must dispose.

HOW IT'S MARKETED: TERMS OF ART

- **Luxury:** usually another way of saying Three-Ply
- **Quilted:** same as Luxury
- **Plush:** same as Quilted
- **Durable:** same as Plush
- **Ultra-Soft:** Three-Ply that is typically NOT Recycled, and potentially contains more bleaching for softening
- **Soft:** normally Two-Ply
- **Absorbent:** same as Soft
- **Strong:** same as Absorbent
- **Environmental:** usually Recycled, sometimes Bamboo
- **Organic/Natural:** usually doesn't contain bleaching or chemical compounds like BPA

CAREFUL CONSIDERATIONS

This is a personal journey—*when you stock your own loo, it's totally up to you.* Rather than give recommendations, here are some things to consider when picking your paper. The three C's:

- **Comfort:** Single-ply may get your fingernails dirty, but three-ply might feel like wiping with a weighted blanket. Everyone has a different range and threshold here.
- **Cost:** An easy way to consistently save is getting off-brand, single-ply toilet paper. If you want more

support with each wipe, go with the bunching technique or fold multiple times.

- **Clogging:** Every home toilet has its own unique flush capacity that must be "felt out" with trial and error. Consider a lower-ply solution if your toilet has fragile pipes.

ALTERNATIVE WIPING OPTIONS (WHEN IN A PINCH)

- **Wet Wipes:** These work for regular and post-wipe work, as well as cleaning the toilet seat of any contraband hairs, dust, sweat, etc. Double-check you are using the flushable kind if that's your intention, as not all are suitable in the plumbing. Contrary to popular belief, they are not great for wiping your face. I still recommend the traditional washcloth there.

- **Napkins/Paper Towels/Tissues:** Gets the job roughly done, but DO NOT flush! These will consistently clog most toilets; they belong in the trash.

- **Sanitary Pads:** Same as above. Okay for wiping, but not for flushing.

- **Wash Cloth/Towel:** If you absolutely must go this route, try to find a Navy or generally dark color. I recommend the trash outside and a trip to the store to replace it.

BRING BACK COLORS!

Most bathrooms now have a modern design, which is conducive to white thrones and toilet paper. But if you are going for a more retro bathroom aesthetic, or just enjoy nostalgia from the '50s, '60s, and '70s, colored toilet paper could be a great addition! They lost popularity in the '80s because it was thought the color-dye chemicals were harmful to your skin, but that has been debunked (most toilet paper is already bleached). If a solid color isn't enough, text and graphics are also available, as well as scented!

POTTY PERFUME

We've already talked about how to avoid smelly bathrooms when going, but as a host you can really provide some assistance here with just a few simple "scentsation" products:

- **Air Fresheners:** They certainly do remove the poop smell after business has been conducted, but they also leave a strong chemical scent. I am not a fan of these.
- **Preemptive Pre-Poo Sprays:** Spray this into the toilet bowl before you deliver the package. It also has a chemical smell, but it's at least more contained to the toilet area.

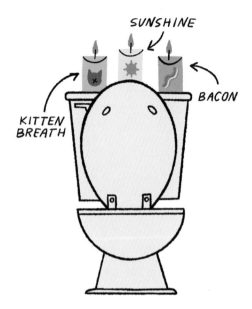

**Choose scents that will transport
you to a happy place.**

- **Matches:** My favorite option. Reminds me of s'mores around a summer campfire. Not for homes with small children!

- **Candles:** Pairs well with matches, with so many scent possibilities. The only way to do this wrong is by picking a bad scent—like "the zoo." Yeah, that actually exists as a candle scent. I love the zoo, but I am certainly not there for the smell. Just make sure to extinguish the candle before leaving home.

TAKING THE PLUNGE

It feels wrong to not let Plungie cover this one.

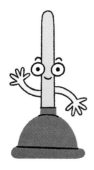

(Plungie takes the typewriter away.) Wow, thank you! This is such an honor! We plungers are the first responders of the bathroom, the paramedics for your emergencies! We come in three main types: Cup, Flange, and Accordion. With regards to toilets, I always recommend the Flange plunger because it has an extra flap to create complete suction on the drain. The Cup plunger is best for sinks, and the Accordion is a just bit harder to get to create a seal (that's why they are usually the grumpiest).

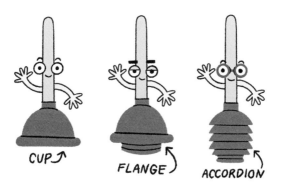

No matter which type you have, make sure to always plunge us straight up and down (I'm talking perpendicular to the floor) instead of at an angle toward your body. And when our rubber starts to show wear and tear, you know it's time for a replacement. We really appreciate a rinse afterward too so that we're ready for the next emergency!

That reminds me of this one time when I was working at a Taco Bell bathroom and—

(The typewriter is quickly recovered from Plungie.)

FLUSHER FIX-UPS

Most toilets have a total lifetime of around thirty to fifty years, so they were outliving humans up until the turn of the twentieth century.[35] Just like cars, there's upkeep required to keep your throne in shape. Here are some common issues beyond the obvious clog that may require a plumbing professional to fix:

- **Leaks:** Your toilet uses quite a few seals, so if you notice water collecting on the floor around it, most likely one has broken.
- **Slow Bowl Draining:** This usually points to a clog somewhere deeper in the pipes. Wire hangers can be helpful here to unhook the buildup in the pipe.
- **Tank Trickling:** This annoying noise could suggest several components are malfunctioning in the tank (float, refill tube, ballcock, or inlet valve).

---

35 In 1905, the human life expectancy became 51 years, officially dethroning the throne.

- **Phantom Flush:** This spooky situation is when the toilet flushes without any use. These are usually caused by a bad flapper valve.

And here are some simple things you can do to try to help your toilet out a bit:

- **Water Softeners:** Using a water softener system at home will help prevent the buildup of calcium in your toilet piping, which causes leaks and clogs.
- **Tank Testing:** Open the lid and perform a flush. Your fill valve should stop dispensing once the water has reached the previous fill line again.
- **Kill Switch Valve:** The shut-off valve (usually found behind the toilet) is the gatekeeper for water getting to the pipes. This should easily turn on and off. If the switch is resistant, this is also a sign something is wrong.

THE PORCELAIN PERCH

If you happen to find yourself in the toilet seat market,[36] don't just select the standard seat—have your butt bucket be a custom retreat for your cheeks. Make sure the shape of the seat suits your behind (behind shapes are more

36 No judgment on whatever happened to your old toilet seat.

different than you think), so do some sitting recon when out and about:

- **Round:** the standard circle seat
- **Elongated (Oval):** the more modern look, a bit bigger than the round one
- **Square:** for a different design and shape appeal
- **D-Shaped:** a combination of square and elongated, this shape has emerged on the scene recently
- **Octagon:** some people like sitting on a stop sign
- **Star:** everyone deserves to feel special!

If you want different material design, you have options besides the standard plastic seat:

- **Wood:** Make Ron Swanson proud by becoming more one with the woods.
- **Shaggy/Fuzzy:** What a nice tribute to the '70s! This can be excellent for a themed party. I can't recommend this from a cleanliness perspective, though, or if you live somewhere extremely hot.[37] Goes well with carpeted bathroom floors.
- **Clear:** These transparent seats are great if you are going for an "under the sea" themed bathroom, as they normally have fish, shells, and basically the whole Great Barrier Reef of objects inside them. Great for a kid's bathroom or a beach house!

---

37 You're in dangerous butt sweat territory.

(ASK PLUNGIE)

Water Closet Wonders

Which facilities sit atop the throne of thrones as the biggest of them all? There are two clear winners here, in two different ways:

- **Functional, by square footage:** In Ichihara City, about an hour drive outside Tokyo,[38] this public restroom is actually a tourist destination because it's basically a private poop garden. This public bathroom is a transparent glass stall (think magician's escape box) surrounded by a 200-square-meter garden, which makes it the biggest, most peaceful "quiet place" of them all.

- **Conceptual, in sheer size:** The biggest toilet based on toilet bowl width and depth, this monumental monstrosity is part of the kidcommons children's museum in Columbus, Indiana. The toilet bowl is the beginning of a slide, if you ever wanted to experience the point of view of your poop as it gets flushed away.

---

38 Tokyo is also home to a "poop museum," an entertaining and aesthetically pleasing place (classic Japan) centered on, well, toilets and turds. The Unko Museum has interactive and intelligence spaces to learn more about pooping (my dream). More on Japan later!

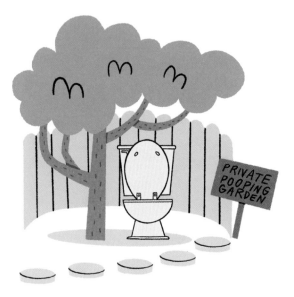

The hills are alive with the sound of flushing.

TOILET STOOLS (BOWEL BOOSTERS)

No, not that kind of stool—a seat for your feet! This toilet elevator is an essential item in your bathroom if you have trouble going or if you sit on the toilet a while before you go. The poop platform helps change your posture on the toilet to simulate a squat, which straightens out your bowels and colon, and lets things flow more naturally.[39] A common analogy is that sitting on the toilet is like putting a kink in your internal hose (colon), but squatting or

39 Less straining on the toilet means you're less likely to suffer from hemorrhoids, which you are mathematically certain to be happier living without.

using a stool straightens the hose back out for better flow. This was proven in studies!

MATS AMORE

Everybody should have a cushy floor mat in front of the commode. Not only are they a delicious treat for your feet (instead of ice-cold tile), but they keep you from slipping in the splash zone. Falling in the shower is already an issue; don't slip on the way out because the floor is wet, which can be hard to see when there's no slippery-when-wet sign. Optimize your choice for grip, comfort, and color. Memory foam is even available. Like shower curtains, bath mats are customizable, so you can choose your own design or image to print, and they're a great gift (or prank) option for friends and family.

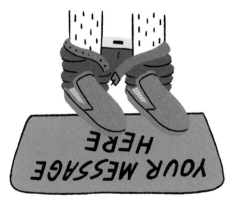

Live! Laugh! Love!

LATHER LOUNGE

Of course, always wash your hands after going. Like toilet paper, it's worth keeping backup supplies. Since you'll be washing after every throne visit, and other times too, don't just grab the cheapest option. Savor the possibilities: organic, moisturizing, scented, soothing, luxurious, hydrating . . . Seriously, you can go nuts in this aisle at many stores. Treat yourself—your hands are worth it!

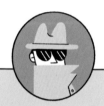

AGENT 002 MISSION

Spice Up Your Sh*t Life

You are bonded for life with your home toilet, and sometimes a commitment of that length can create a dull relationship. Your mission now is to appreciate your pooping partner. Here are a few ways to keep things exciting in your relationship.

- **New Seat, Who Dis:** The glue that connects you both together = a fresh seat.
- **No Phone:** Taking in the moment every once in a while creates a more connected experience.
- **Open Relationship:** Get more experience pooping in public so that when you come

home you feel more appreciative of who's waiting for you.

- **New Shine (Cleaning):** A little prep might make you both feel better for the next time.
- **New Gadgets:** Double-ply toilet paper, new decorations, new bath mat—all of these help create a more enjoyable experience.
- **Laxatives:** This is the most bold, but you will certainly appreciate your toilet after this.
- **Leave the Door Open:** For the potential thrill of being caught, even if you live alone!
- **Couples Commode:** An additional adjacent toilet so you and your lover can share the shituary together at home.

All relationships take effort. Your toilet time isn't any different.

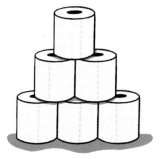

TRICKING OUT THE THRONE ROOM, PART TWO: THE FUN STUFF

WHAT YOUR LOO SAYS ABOUT YOU

Your home bathroom should be a sanctuary where you can recharge and escape the stresses of daily life. If hosting relatives for the holidays becomes too much, or you simply want to swipe through some cat videos in peace, the bathroom is your solitude sanctuary. Whether you want to dream, read, listen, scroll, or just close your eyes for a moment, your bathroom should maximize these benefits to give you the best experience! A simple way to start that shift is crafting your space to curate the mood you desire. The bathroom is a no-pressure place to fully express your inner style and artistic desires,[40] so let's get to it!

THE ROCK-OUT REFUGE

Create some audio ambience with a little private concert venue. Singing outside the shower is socially acceptable,

---

40 Go for it! As long as it contains a toilet, you're good!

especially if you are still in the bathroom. A smaller room with close walls offers excellent reverb.

Essentials: Bluetooth speaker, mood lighting, microphone

Next Level: stage lighting, floor amps, small instruments, dry ice smoke

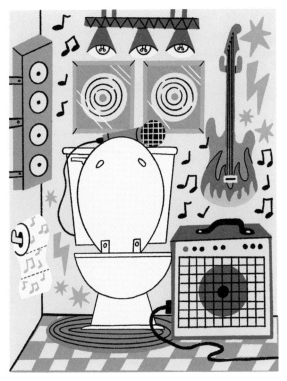

Turn it up!

THE RELAXING RETREAT

A stress-free self-care center, this is a mini "treat yourself" corner that you can visit daily—you deserve it!

Essentials: dimmed light, incense, candles, calming music, phone stand (hands free)[41]

Next Level: Gaia-energy-giving plants,[42] peaceful mural or wallpaper, starscape projected on the ceiling, actual grass mat to feel between your toes

THE COLLECTOR'S CORNER

The bathroom is a judgment-free zone, and a place that provides a natural focus of attention. There's no better place to appreciate the self-expression of your collection.

Essentials: Beanie Babies, taxidermy, creepy dolls, bobbleheads (whatever your jam is, but lots of them)

Next Level: Add collection-customized shower curtains, toilet seat covers, posters, nightlights, mirror frames—go crazy.

THE READING ROOM

Screen-free entertainment can also be a nice change of pace, and bathroom books are a great way to do that.[43]

Essentials: Hella books. Anything that's not serving as a bookcase is wasted space.

---

41   Helps you avoid the stress of accidentally dropping your phone in the toilet!
42   I recommend a bonsai tree here (if it can be kept inside).
43   I hear bathroom books are really on the rise, especially one in particular . . .

Next Level: cozy sweater, directional reading lights, tea kettle, a cat

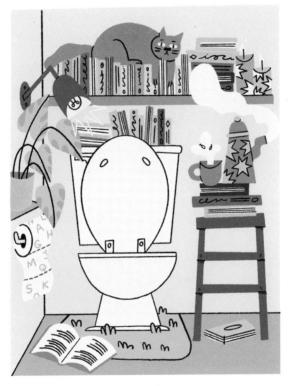

A quiet place.

THE GAMER'S GROTTO

Real gamers know that bathroom breaks cut into high scores. Take a break between activities with a quick session, or use this as a natural way to limit your gaming time if you're trying to cut it down these days.

Essentials: headphones or speaker, game system of choice, monitor, strong Wi-Fi

Next Level: custom toilet seat gamer chair, multiple monitors, Hot Pockets, bowl of Skittles, surround sound speakers

THE QUIET CUBE

An isolation chamber is the perfect place to forget the world for a moment and use your bathroom as a con-templation capsule to go on an inner journey. A brief reclusive retreat.

Essentials: noise-cancelling headphones, lights out, eyes closed, neck pillow

Next Level: everything painted black, soundproofed walls, blackout curtains, light-blocking door trim

THE THRONE ROOM

Give yourself the medieval aristocratic treatment.

Essentials: crown, gilded toilet, robe, champagne, grapes, a footstool with a cushion

Next Level: scepter, suit of armor, bejeweled shower curtain, toilet paper dispensed from gryphon's head

BEACH MODE (UNDER THE SEA)

Sometimes you can't book a flight to get away, but you can still find your beach if you have a nautical-themed throne room. Have a coastal view from the crapper!

Essentials: tropical wallpaper, beach towels, *Finding Nemo* shower curtain

Next Level: sunscreen, beach ball, lobster hand towel, sea turtles on the ceiling

Thar she blows!

Throne of Thrones—
Royal Restroom Edition

You might assume that royal status would not spare
one from some of the toilet practicalities common to
all, but you would be wrong. Consider the more private throne-room life of King Henry XIII—he did not
even wipe himself. That task was performed by the
Groom of the Stool, also called the Chief Gentleman
of the Chamber. He was responsible for setting up
the toilet, removing the king's valuables before he
did his business, talking to him, wiping the king,
and cleaning the station. Weirdly, people actually
really wanted this position because it had so much
intimate time with the king. Henry also had hot
and cold water taps in his bathroom, which was
rare in the 1500s (which is sometimes still true
in my apartment building today).

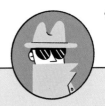

AGENT 002 MISSION

Night Crawling

(In a hushed whispering tone)

It's quiet hours, which means stealth mode has been activated. Whether that last glass of water got you out of bed or you were burning the midnight oil, it's time to use the toilet (quietly). You want to avoid fully waking your sleeping partner still in bed, or even worse, disturbing someone else sleeping in the house. There are two main sources of sensory input that wake a sleeping person—light and noise. Because you are at home, you should know this bathroom like the back of your hand. Try to maneuver with just a night-light[44] or even your phone's flashlight. If you've got a toilet that screams as a flusher, consider leaving the waste there until morning.[45]

---

44 They also keep the monsters away—adults are also afraid of the dark!
45 What's that saying? If it's brown, flush it down; if it's yellow, let it mellow.

GREAT ESCAPES: HOME EDITION

Even at home, the bathroom sometimes is the only place in the house where you can lock the door, turn on some tunes, and pretend that the rest of the world doesn't exist. Sure, you may hear the faint knocking of a family member or roommate, or the door scritching of devoted pets, but that's why we have noise-cancelling headphones. It's like a mini-vacation from reality, a place where you can sit on the porcelain throne and reign supreme. So next time you need a break from your loved ones or roommates, you don't need to book a flight, just head to the bathroom for a bit and let your troubles be flushed away—and come back to the living area ready and recharged.

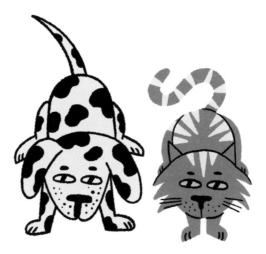

Pets may want to share this special time with you.

THE BIDET: BEYOND WIPING

It's time to bring out the white tablecloth, because you're now entering the ToiletPlus[46] section of the bathroom. And like any good Michelin-starred prix fixe, everything is taken care of for you, starting with the pre-warmed seat. This toilet feels like soiling on a cloud, including a hands-free, no-wiping experience. If you have trouble waking up in the morning, you'll certainly appreciate the fountain technology that can send a cool, clean splash right up there. It's booty bliss.

WHAT IS IT?

While it sounds fancy, a bidet is just a station, usually found in the bathroom, that's used to clean one's private parts.[47] The cleaning is provided by a water faucet spray action that you sit on, similar to a toilet. The main types:

- **Conventional/Freestanding:** This is a separate station from the toilet and is not flushable for defecating. Looks like an empty bowl with just a sink faucet head.
- **Shower:** These attach to the wall and can be moved around like a hose or shower head, so standing works great. You might want to do this in a tub or floor area with a drain, though.

---

46 Unlike many other "plus" services, this one doesn't come with a monthly subscription fee.
47 Cleaning feet is actually another common usage, and they are arguably much dirtier and more visible. Next time you see a bidet, give your feet a look.

- **Add On/Integrated:** This one attaches to a toilet, usually on the back rim or the seat, and creates a two-for-one station where you can use a traditional toilet with additional bidet features.

HOW DOES IT WORK?

Instead of using paper products to clean our butt area after defecating, this method instead applies water pressure to freshen up and clean your cheeks. In most cases, this makes toilet paper optional, which is better for the environment, cheaper, and sometimes even more effective.[48]

Also, yes, you can usually control the water pressure and temperature. So it doesn't have to be a shock but a soothing rinse.

HOLD UP, IS IT BETTER FOR THE ENVIRONMENT?

Bidets are a triple threat to saving the planet: They reduce toilet paper waste (approximately fifteen million trees a year), save water (37 gallons used per roll of TP), and avoid exposing the environment to harsh chemicals like bleach and formaldehyde. So, not only are bidets better for your booty, they're also a win for the planet in pretty much every way.

---

48 It is actually quite hard to prove that your butt is cleaner using a bidet vs traditional paper wiping, but the argument commonly used is, "If you walked outside barefoot in the grass and stepped on a pile of dog poop, would you clean your feet using only dry napkins?"

OKAY, SO WHERE ARE THEY FOUND?

I mean, everywhere. They've been around since the 1700s and in some countries are even required alongside public toilets (hello, Portugal). Most credit Japan for making bidets universally popular, but they really have been popular throughout Europe and Asia for decades.

HOW CAN I GET ONE?

For the traditional freestanding bidet, your bathroom needs to be inspected by a professional to make sure you have the space and proper water piping for one. Then you can expect to pay anywhere from a few hundred to a few thousand dollars for product and installation.

For bidet beginners, the toilet seat attachment is a great way to dip your toes into the technology.[49] They just attach to your current seat or replace it with a new bidet-integrated seat. Most models cost a few hundred dollars.

JAPANESE TOILET TECHNOLOGY

Speaking of Japan, welcome to the future, where even your toilet is now sentient. But don't be afraid of all the buttons—these super toilets are amazing. They commonly include built-in features like a bidet (see above), deodorization, seat warming, white noise generation, water

49 Well, more like your tushy than toes.

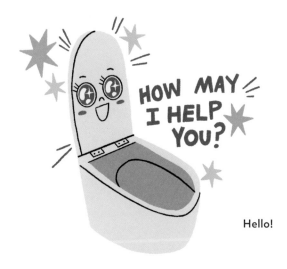

HOW MAY I HELP YOU?

Hello!

pressure/temperature control, blow-drying, self-cleaning, and auto-flushing. Even glow-in-the-dark seats for night-time mode! Trust me, the motion-detection technology is accurate; they auto-opened every time I was even near my bathroom when visiting Japan, which caused quite a few startles during my middle-of-the-night sessions.[50] But arguably the most impressive part about these toilets is that they aren't just for the rich and famous: **80 percent of Japanese households have these advanced smart seats**, as do most public bathrooms, restaurants, and hotels.

There are rumors that even a "medical toilet" is in the works, one that measures your blood sugar from urine

---

50 I'm not against good customer service, but sometimes overattentiveness can be a bit creepy. Let me lift my own seat when ready, especially when suffering from extreme jet lag!

and stools, and even the blood pressure and body fat of the user. Connected to the Internet, these online toilets can alert a doctor upon uncommon or dangerous findings. Voice commands are also being experimented with, so maybe one day we will be talking to our toilet!

Besides the toilet tech, I've never seen a place that has so many accessible (and clean) public restroom options. I'm talking convenient stores, gas stations, restaurants, malls, parks, you name it. The United States can and should do better here.

THE FUTURE OF FLUSHING

Everybody dreams of a future where society works together seamlessly and issues like war, poverty, and world hunger disappear. Here's what I hope the facilities end up being in our future.

TOILET WHISPERER

Is your toilet acting naughty? Does it rebelliously refuse to flush in the most random ways? It might be time to call a *Toilet Whisperer* for help! These highly trained experts can listen to your toilet *grrrp* and *blrrrp* for a bit and then instantly repair the root of your broken relationship. We also offer family counseling services in case multiple parties in your household are having trouble with the toilet! Just call 1-800-MY-TOILET-MATTERS.

TOILET PAPER GENIE

Have you ever been so desperate in a wiping position that the new towel from Bed Bath & Beyond becomes your best bet? Tired of delicately tiptoeing to your car looking for extra fast-food napkins when you're completely out of stock? Well, say goodbye to that and hello to the *TP Genie*, who can be easily summoned by just rubbing the cardboard tube from your empty roll. These genies always have double- and triple-ply ready for you, even in shipping shortages!

BATHROOM SWAG ALARM

Annoyed by people barging into your unlocked bathroom? Tired of looking sweaty emerging from a bathroom with no air-conditioning? Or do you have nightmares about leaving the bathroom with toilet paper stuck to your shoe? Fear no more! When the *Swag Alarm* is installed, the bathroom auto-locks after entering and won't let you leave until you freshen (fix) your appearance for the waiting world! Now you won't ever accidentally leave the bathroom again looking like a . . . well, just not your best self.

iTOILET

From the company that has brought you the iPad, iPhone, and the iCar, we proudly present the *iToilet*. Not only do these toilets come in sleek black and white designs, but they also support VaporPlay and have chargers ready so you can juice on the john. It's a hands-free experience, as the toilet can be locked and unlocked with facial recognition technology, so your personal privy is protected. But that's not all—if you ever drop your ear pods in the toilet (oh, you will), the *iToilet* will immediately replace them with a new pair! You can just leave the dropped buds in the bowl and they will be automatically disposed of in ways we can't legally explain in writing![51]

NOISE-CANCELLING TOILETS

Are you sick and tired of your neighbors hearing your heinie horn? Or are you a parent who's always exhausted because your "noises" keep waking up your napping newborn? Did you recently read a bathroom book that classified you as an Announcer-type-toilet-user type but then gave you bogus advice like play music and run the sink to simulate white noise? Well, we have the perfect toilet for you—an oasis of peace and quiet—a toilet that prevents any sound created on it from escaping! Crap with confidence knowing that nobody's day will be ruined by you anymore.

---

51 Does this experience feel too real? No worries at all because the iToilet is also supported in AR/VR through a simple (but *expensive*) headset. Experience the joy of using the throne from the comfort of your couch or anywhere you like for just a few thousand dollars.

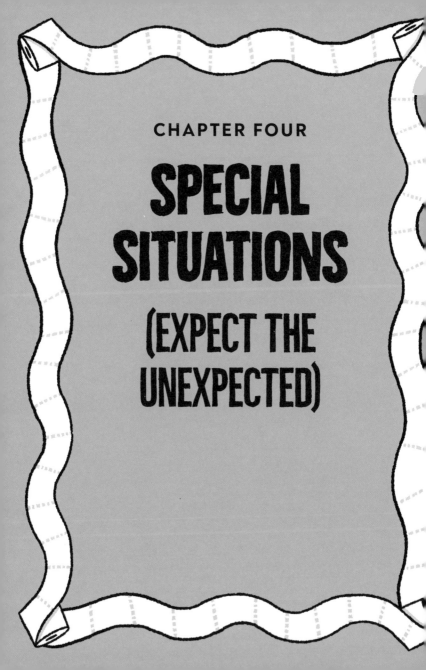

CHAPTER FOUR

SPECIAL SITUATIONS (EXPECT THE UNEXPECTED)

PLANES, TRAINS, AND TURBULENT TOILETING

Confined spaces, long lines, aisles, seating situations, and fellow passengers to navigate: these special circumstances need strategic approaches.

- **Before Takeoff:** Try to reserve an aisle seat if you're a "goer," but feel no shame or compunction about excusing yourself and politely getting out from your middle or window seat. Everyone's got to go, and you'd do the same for someone else.
- **Layer Down:** Remove bulky clothing items for flexibility (jackets, sleeves) but have your shoes on—lots of people take them off on long trips. These bathrooms tend to be tiny, so giants and professional athletes take special note of this one.[52]
- **Make It Count:** It takes a bit of effort to get to these toilets and they are usually in high demand, so make sure you've finished all your business on this precious trip.

52 I'm actually 6'4", but unfortunately not a professional athlete, until using the bathroom becomes a sport.

- **Close the Lid:** Always good advice, but especially on airplanes—they have jet-engine-power-flushing capabilities.
- **Skip Courtesy Flush:** It gets the hopes up of those waiting, and you don't need to worry about clogging anyways (see bullet above).
- **Stretch:** While waiting in line, move around. These are rare moments of relief.
- **Stay Hydrated:** Some avoid drinking water during travel to limit bathroom breaks. On planes, however, you're already dehydrating faster than usual (cabins are kept at 10 to 20 percent humidity compared to a more normal 35 to 65 percent). Especially on a longer flight, hydrate and be bold about using the bathroom.

⇨ **RANDOM SHORT RANT** ☺
SHAKES ON A PLANE

What's the deal with turbulence always seeming to strike when I'm standing up from my seat on a bathroom break? Turbulence on the toilet always feels like a severe weather situation, like I'm starring in *Shakes on a Plane*—the real-life sequel to *Snakes on a Plane*.

ASK PLUNGIE

What Happens to Our Waste?

Planes: It's *not* ejected into the air midflight as "blue ice," as exciting as that myth may be. It's stored safely in a tank and pumped out by a service trunk upon landing.

Trains: Historically, this waste was dumped in transit, right on the tracks! These days they keep it tanked up like in planes. Trains in the Netherlands and Switzerland go one better and employ self-composting toilets, which only need to be emptied twice a year.

Ships: Sadly, ships still dump their waste into the ocean, especially when over international waters and from older models with no sewage tanks. Modern cruise ships have sanitation farms that separate the waste from the water before dumping back into the ocean. Recently, marine technology has been focused on preventing as much ocean pollution as possible.[53]

---

53 It's getting really bad—just google "great pacific garbage patch" if you are okay with feeling a little sad.

⇨ **RANDOM SHORT RANT** ☺
GETTING OUT OF THE AISLE

Have you ever noticed how asking a stranger to let you out to use the bathroom on a plane or train feels like you're asking for a kidney transplant? It's like you're inconveniencing them beyond belief by daring to have bodily functions. And don't even get me started on the gymnastics required to climb over your seatmate when they're asleep. Can't we all just agree to normalize asking to be let out to use the toilet!

SPACE

You just never know where you might find yourself. Luckily, you must be specially trained for how to go in space, positioning yourself in relation to the bowl and using leg restraints to stay in place. The system has been engineered so that a vacuum system is running the entire time you are in the chamber, so that solid and liquid wastes are collected in the bowl right away, without floating away in zero-gravity conditions. The liquid wastewater is released into the void, and the solid is stored in little bags.

In 2020, a new space toilet was developed called Universal Waste Management System that finally does a better job of factoring female anatomy into the design, because the urine funnel and seat can now be used simultaneously.

GREAT ESCAPES: SPECIAL SITUATIONS EDITION

Ah, the airplane lavatory, a tiny oasis of tranquility amid the chaos of air travel. It's the one place on a plane where you can shut out the world, even if just for a few minutes. And let's not forget about the train or bus bathroom, where you can escape the cramped quarters and stretch your legs (or just your arms, depending on the size of the bathroom). Even out in nature, the bathroom can be a welcome respite from the elements. Just find a secluded spot, dig a little hole, and voila! Whether you're exploring new lands or just in transit, the bathroom can always provide a brief moment of solace.

(GOING) ON THE ROAD AGAIN

You only have two thousand more miles to go when the feeling always hits. Stuck in the middle of nowhere, the car is full of gas, but now so are you. Here's what I look for when deciding if this next exit is *my exit* to empty out:

- First off, it's recommended you stop every two to three hours (one hundred miles) for a fifteen-minute stretch, so pair that with your bathroom or snack breaks. A double date with you and the loo.

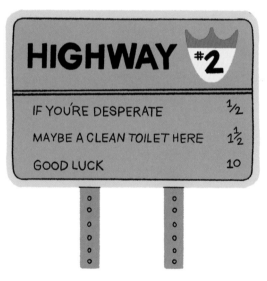

Choose wisely.

- Ideally, try NOT to steer off the highway to a place that has just the one gas station/shack that probably every desperate soul has used. With more options, you'll have a chance for an actually not-bad experience, and won't have to go in a hole out back if *Dave's Deserted Last-Chance Gas 'n' Guzzles* crapper is out of commission.

- It's okay to pay to play here. Road trips have special rules where everyone needs to take breaks from driving with very unhealthy but morale-boosting nostalgic snacks. So consider the edible options at the restaurant or gas station. You might be hungry afterward,[54] and usually there's a correlation between good food and clean restrooms.

- Please do a double take at the sink when washing your hands to make sure all crevices are covered! Road-trip restrooms commonly host bacteria meet and greets.

It's a great feeling getting back in your car with a full tank of gas and an empty colon, ready to rock the rest of your trip!

---

54 I eat so much when driving all day. Ankle movement burns so many calories—really a total-body workout including the steering too.

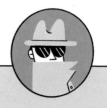

AGENT 002 MISSION

Worst Toilet Times Tight Five

As a field agent, you will be put in stressful situations when on assignments. Your mission is to successfully navigate using the bathroom in what I've found to be the Tight Five of Worst Toilet Times. Proceed with caution:

- **The Fair:** Have you seen what people eat at fairs?[55] And then the situation they put their stomachs in by riding the *SpinDaddy 360* afterward? The bathrooms are crowded, dirty, and full of folks in critical conditions.

- **The Club:** The last thing you want to do when drunk is to take care of business. Intoxicated stall neighbors are unpredictable—the situation can go very north or south in an instant. It's also weird to feel the house music vibrate the toilet seat.

- **First Date:** Every move you make matters. After all, this is an interview with some sexual tension (hopefully). Even when the date is back at home, every moment is critical for you to put on a show. Disappearing for long stretches is just not in the success playbook.

55   Hint: It's all deep fried. Even the water fountains.

- **Formal Occasions**: The issue here is not the bathrooms being nice but you wanting to look nice. Taking off a formal dress or tuxedo, making a deposit, and then redonning your attire just never looks quite the same. You get one shot before getting dressed, and then you have to ride it out the rest of the night. Appearance is the priority.
- **Standardized Testing**: These dumb timed tests can decide your whole future, so every second literally drains your presidential potential. This applies to the SAT, ACT, Driving Test, GMAT, LSAT, MCAT, and BuzzFeed's "Which Hogwarts House Do You Belong In?"

WHEN NATURE CALLS

Yes, some of you will even find yourself here, bonding with nature during a vulnerable moment just like our ancestors did every day. I assume anyone in this situation is at their breaking point, so just be bold and, as they say, *let it go*. I've actually only used nature's toilet once, and it was certainly . . . not a success. So to offer you actual expert advice, I turn the mic over to Dirty Mike, who dropped out of college to hike the Appalachian Trail (about 2,200 miles) and then did the Colorado Trail (about 575 miles) after graduating.

HOW MANY TIMES HAVE YOU USED NATURE'S TOILET?

It's safe to say I've used it five hundred plus times. They don't call me Dirty Mike for nothing.

WALK US THROUGH HOW TO EXECUTE IT SUCCESSFULLY.

It obviously requires a little more forethought than plopping down on an old porcelain throne. Hip flexibility is important because you need to be able to do a deep squat. First, you need to find toilet paper. My tool of choice is a clump of long grass and a few smooth sticks, but this is going to depend on what vegetation is growing in your environment. Find a grassy patch and pull two to three handfuls, depending on how messy you predict it to be. As for sticks, make sure to find some that are about the diameter of your index finger and have smooth bark for comfort. Now that you have your materials, it's time to find a spot to do the deed, so look for a flat or slightly sloped surface and a small tree to hold on to for stability. Take your sticks and dig a nice big shit-sized hole, do your deep squat above, and let her rip—you'll be surprised how easily it will flow out. Don't be too hard on yourself if you miss your target; you can scoop the mess into the hole after (cue the sticks). Sometimes I like to put a nice rock on top of my hole as a capstone. I usually go grass wipe first, then two stick wipes, finishing off with one last grass wipe. Put your pants back on and continue your adventure, hopefully with a slightly lighter pack!

WORST SITUATION YOU'VE ENCOUNTERED?

One day in the mountains of North Carolina, we were experiencing a freezing rainstorm, where it was turning to ice in our hair and on our clothes. On this day, one of my hiking partners was starting to feel sick. In his weakened state, he felt a shitstorm coming. He picked an innocent tree to hold and did his squat when—BAM!—the tree broke and he fell straight into his own poop. Let me just say, there was not enough Purell in a two-ounce canister to take care of that mess.

SIGNIFICANCE BEHIND THE *LEAVE NO TRACE* PHILOSOPHY?

Picture this: You are one with nature in the wilderness, amazed by its beauty and grandeur, when suddenly you see a clump of used toilet paper on the ground. And then another one. And then another one. No one wants to see or smell that. We share the woods with wildlife and every other hiker who comes after us. Bury your shit, and if you use toilet paper, bury it extra deep![56]

---

56 All toilet paper is actually biodegradable, but depending on conditions, it can take up to three years to fully decompose. That's why burying it is so critical, or you can buy specific toilet paper made to dissolve faster in nature, which can reduce the total decomposition time down to one month.

General Rule of Thumb: Bury six to eight inches deep, at least two hundred feet from water, and cover up the hole with whatever you can find.

WHAT IF YOU CAN'T GO ON THE GROUND AT ALL?

This is called *Pack it in, pack it out*. If you are hiking in a high alpine area, you will not be able to go on the ground. Especially if it's high traffic. Those areas simply can't handle it. This was the case when we hiked Mount Whitney (Sierra Nevada, California). We took a "go" bag and hoped that we wouldn't have to go. Unfortunately, one of my partners was having stomach issues and had to use the same bag three times. The bag was pretty full.

GENERAL TOOLS & TIPS

- Stick your butt out as far as possible to make sure the waterfall trajectory has enough clearance from your pants and shoes.
- Make sure your back is facing civilization, and not your front. *The moon is much easier to look at than the sun.*
- The shit shovel is for digging the hole, not for shoveling your stools. Don't let it touch the poop at all, or it becomes unsanitary and needs to be stored separately.

- Wiping Hierarchy: Grass > Smooth Sticks > Snow > Stones > Leaves
  - » Snow can make great toilet paper. Bunch it up into a snowball and it will melt a little while you use it, just like a bidet.
  - » A smooth river stone is also a great wiping alternative. It is structurally very sound, so you can put a lot of force behind it.
  - » Stay away from leaves. They don't do well with shear stress; you can poke a finger through easily!
  - » Check for bugs on the "toilet paper"—every side of the surface!
- DO NOT FORGET to bury the evidence or pack it back out. You want to preserve the beauty and stifle the scent, which hopefully won't attract animals to it.

For more information on safely disposing in the wilderness, check out LNT.org.

TECHNICAL DIFFICULTIES

OOPS!

Everybody, at some point, will poop their pants. We all did as toddlers, some may again as adults, and we certainly will as senior citizens. Even if it's just a small amount like the shart. *The Great Bowel Movement* usually happens without warning, sometimes as a one-off accident, and other times it's due to fecal incontinence, where one cannot physically stop the urge to defecate. Let's remove the shame behind a completely natural occurrence and focus on the sanitary solution for it.

No time is a good time to have a bowel accident, but being at home makes it much easier. Ditch the underwear in a trash can OUTSIDE. Give the trousers a rinse down and then a solo wash. Do not make the mistake of putting poopy pants in the laundry hamper and washing with other garments. That is gross.

On the go is a different story. Find a bathroom (standalone is best) as quickly as possible to assess damage. Ditch the undergarments in the bathroom trash can. If your pants are in decent shape, it's time to rock commando the rest of the day. If not, clean as much as you can with paper towels, soap, and water from the sink, and then try to get home ASAP. Throw away the pants. It's officially okay to cancel the rest of your commitments that day—you survived a very stressful situation.

THE RUNS ON A RUN

It's extremely common to experience *runner's gut* (the strong urge to go during a run). Over half the running population reports having needed to pause for a poop break. This happens for a couple of reasons:

- Blood is flowing to your muscles instead of your GI tract, which is responsible for absorbing water down there to slow down the flow.
- Making lots of movement also causes disruptions in your GI tract, making you more likely to go.

Here's a few things you can do to limit runner's stomach and dodge this issue altogether:

- Stick to eating carbohydrates, which are easier to digest.
- Avoid fatty and high-protein foods, caffeine, and sugary sweets.
- Plan your pre-run poops.

PHONING IT IN

Doom scrollers beware: Dropping your phone in the toilet happens to 20 percent of cell phone users. Most phones are water resistant these days, so you don't need to worry about sticking it into rice or cat litter overnight to remove moisture (unless you've got an older phone, circa 2015), but you should give it a thorough cleaning to avoid bacteria aftershock. This can be done with cotton swabs and rubbing alcohol, or sanitizing wet wipes, but turn off your device before you begin! Your phone is already the biggest germ spreader you touch every day, so this outcome is another reason to leave it in your pocket while pooping.

YOU'RE WEARING A ONESIE

Or a romper, overalls, formal wear, a clown costume, a Santa suit, giant barbarian rabbit cosplay—hey, no judgment here. Fashion over function. Just be especially thorough in checking your layers of stall security *and* make sure you check for a door hook before undoing your duds.

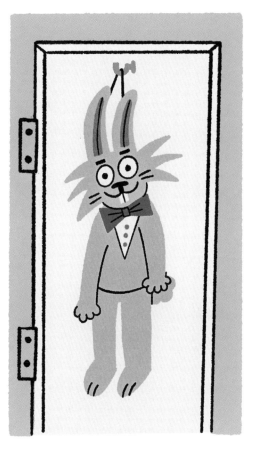

Check for a door hook before
removing difficult clothing.

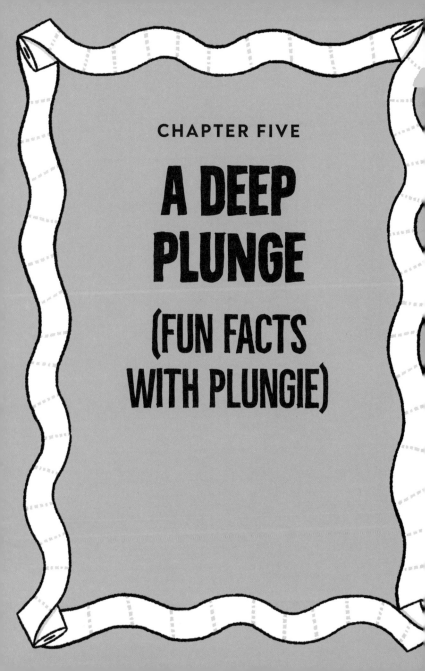

CHAPTER FIVE

A DEEP PLUNGE

(FUN FACTS WITH PLUNGIE)

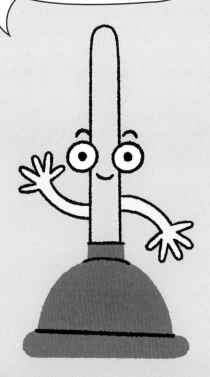

GETTING THINGS MOVING

This whole book we've assumed things are flowing, maybe even more than you'd prefer, but what about when your colon is moving like concrete? I've got your back even when you're backed up. Here are some simple steps to clean out your colon!

- **Drink Water:** Dehydration is a big contributor to constipation.
- **Eat Fiber:** This makes your stool bigger and softer, which is easier to pass. Foods generally rich in fiber include whole-grain breads, beans, vegetables, and fresh fruit. The yummy stuff. Especially PRUNE JUICE. Give it a shot.
- **Drink Coffee:** It keeps your brain sparking *and* stomach moving by stimulating the muscles in your gut.[57] It makes a great regulator and can jump-start things, but it's also a diuretic, so avoid overdoing it and risking dehydration.
- **Exercise:** Moving your body moves your bowels (see p. 140, (Body) Movement for (Bowel) Movement).
- **Massage:** Apply gentle pressure and movement to your abdomen.

---

57 Your stomach needs its morning coffee before starting its day too.

- **Posture:** Raise your knees above your hips when sitting on the toilet.[58]
- **Pay Your Taxes:** The stress of trying to do this correctly and then summing together the total you owe will certainly make your stomach turn!

If the constipation persists, try taking a light form of laxatives, or better yet, see a doctor.

SLOWING THINGS DOWN

On the other hand, you may be in a bind where you want to go less frequently. If you're in a serious situation where your stomach feels like a washing machine, here are some short-term tips to solidify:

- Eat bland foods such as crackers, rice, potatoes, eggs, and toast. If it's really serious, just stick with BRAT (bananas, rice, apples, toast). They don't aggravate your digestive system and are known to be "binders": They will firm up your stool.
- Avoid coffee, alcohol, fried foods, dairy products, and spicy seasonings.
- Avoid dehydration from overgoing by drinking lots of fluids. Consider broths for meal replacement.[59]

---

58 Another plug for toilet stools and squat toilets, which both do this well. Weirdly, the most common toilet seat positioning is not optimally conducive to how we naturally go.

59 If you are ever concerned about your digestive health, a poop journal might be a good idea for you! Unlike our memories, the log doesn't lie, and you can show the doctor a recent record.

WHAT THE HELL IS A "FODMAP"?

FODMAP is an acronym used to represent a sort of carbohydrate chain that causes diarrhea, gas, bloating, stomach cramps, and general digestive stress for some people. FODMAP (fermentable oligosaccharides, disaccharides, monosaccharides, and polyols) foods include certain types of dairy, beans, lentils, breads, fruits, and vegetables.

A low-FODMAP diet avoids such foods for a while, then slowly reintroduces them one by one to try and pinpoint which food disagrees with your system. This can help steer you toward food choices to keep you on a more even keel.

EAT

Bell peppers
Bok choy
Butter
Carrots
Cucumber
Eggplant
Grapes
Lettuce
Oats
Oil
Oranges
Peanuts
Pineapple
Popcorn
Potatoes
Strawberries
Tofu
Tomatoes
Tortilla chips
Zucchini

AVOID

Apples
Asparagus
Avocadoes
Beans
Blackberries
Bread (gluten-based)
Breaded meat
Cashews
Cherries
Garlic
High-fructose corn syrup
Honey
Mangoes
Milk
Mushrooms
Onion
Peaches
Pears
Pistachios
Watermelon
Yogurt

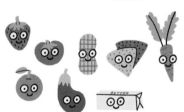

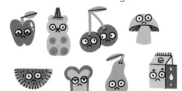

AM I GOING TOO OFTEN? OR NOT OFTEN ENOUGH?

"Normal" is from three times a day to three times a week—which is a pretty wide range of experience! So never mind normal. Do you feel generally comfortable, neither bloated nor urgent, and mostly able to predict when you're likely to go? Your personal consistency matters most here. Some interesting details from a study:[60]

- Half of all people go once a day.
- Almost a third go twice a day.
- Most go in the morning (coffee time), a quarter go in the afternoon (weirdos), and yes, three percent go in the evening (creatures of the night).
- Your digestive tendencies do change as you age, like a lot of things. The most common change is constipation from a loss in muscle tone (time for some crunches), but the other causes above are also in the playing field.

WHY DO WE PEE WHILE WE POOP?

As the saying goes, *Every poo poo is pee pee time, but not all pee pee is poo poo time.* We have smaller muscles that control our pee door, and obviously larger ones that

---

60 Obviously, there are things that shake up your digestion patterns, like all-you-can-eat buffets, traveling, and stuff-your-face holidays. But you should feel like you can predict your patterns during your weekly routine.

open and close our poo gates.[61] When we sit for a poo, we tell the larger muscles controlling that gate to relax, which for most people also involuntarily opens their pee door as well, which is why we pee while waiting for a poo. It is possible to poop without peeing (but this skill is rare), so if that's you, maybe it's time to finally enter that talent show you've been eyeing for years.

DOES FARTING MEAN I HAVE TO POOP?

Not at all! We butt burp to help unload buildup of excess gas in our intestines. This simply could come from drinking too much seltzer or being stressed about something. But you can influence your intestinal gas levels by just modifying your diet (see p. 122, What the Hell Is a "FODMAP"?). Regardless, it's very healthy to get the gas out, and not always a sign of "what's to come" in the bathroom later.

Fun Fact: If you think you fart too much during the day, you should record yourself at night, because the majority of gas gets blown out while we sleep. Your bedmate or dog would have the best insight here.

---

61 The muscle is called a sphincter, which sounds like a medieval weapon. If activated in the right time and place, it can definitely be wielded as one.

WHY DO MY LEGS FALL ASLEEP WHILE ON THE TOILET?

Simply put: nerve compression due to posture (leaned forward, legs bent). Fifteen minutes in this position is usually the threshold for causing that feeling, so those who take their time on the toilet are more at risk. If you want to remove that static feeling in your legs, try to limit your total toilet time (if you can), switch positions every few minutes, strain less, and consider a padded toilet seat. However, if your legs do not wake up a few minutes after getting off the toilet, or are consistently numb, go see a doctor.

WIPING WARS—WHAT'S THE BEST WAY?

Something so universally natural and necessary can weirdly be done in many different ways. This contributes to the argument that using the toilet is in fact a creative art form, but still begs the ultimate better bathroom debate—*what's the right way to wipe?*

STANDING VS SITTING

As a sitter, I've always heard of standers but never understood their position. But the most shocking thing I learned from researching this topic is that almost half of the population stands, so I guess I do know many people in that camp. But alas, the disappointing answer to this spicy question is that there is no "best" way to wipe, so just do whatever feels right to you.[62] Neither form has an advantage in terms of cleanliness or effectiveness. There are even some maniacs who mix it up and bat both ways.[63]

TL;DR: Most sit, but it's *almost* an even split. The rivalry will continue to rage on.

FOLDING VS SCRUNCHING

Another technique people are passionate about, with very little sympathy for the other side. If saving paper is your goal, then folding is the clear choice—folders use half the toilet paper of scrunchers on each wipe. Scrunchers think their technique is more sanitary (bunching your paper into a wad lets it wipe every little crevice) because a neat flat square doesn't fit the shape of our turd cutter sometimes. Men are more likely to fold, while women scrunch. I'm a man, but I like to scrunch, so don't let that stereotype define your wiping technique.

FRONT TO BACK VS BACK TO FRONT

Regardless of preference, there *is* a winner here, and it's *front to back*. That approach moves feces away from your delicate parts with each wipe, reducing risk of cross con- tamination and infection. This is less of a worry for men,

62 Which, if that's standing, is wrong.
63 A Switch-Wiper.

but still a pretty serious consideration for all our wipers out there.

HOW OFTEN SHOULD I CLEAN MY TOILET?

This really depends on how frequently you destroy it. Even though cleanliness is subjective, in order to prevent harmful bacteria growth, you should at least do a light wipe down of your toilet surfaces once a week. Other areas can go longer, but for obvious reasons, the toilet is the final boss of bathroom bacteria buildup.

IT'S THE TWENTY-FIRST CENTURY: CAN'T ROBOTS CLEAN MY TOILET?

This is a safe space to admit that cleaning the toilet sucks. *New York Post* reported on a study ranking it as the "most hated chore in America."[64] If you want to significantly reduce this responsibility, invest in a self-cleaning toilet. It's a specially designed toilet that self-cleans the bowl (typically triggered by a button), which takes care of the most elbow-greasing part.[65] These toilets are obviously a bit more expensive than the standard, but there are cheaper versions that cost only a few hundred dollars.

64 Here are the others: cleaning the oven, cleaning windows, removing hair from the drain (my personal favorite), unclogging the sink. Classic *New York Post* insight.
65 Self-cleaning toilet manufacturers still recommend a general wipe down of the seats and toilet surfaces.

The self-cleaning functionality typically comes with a deodorizer, so your (self-cleaned) toilet should always be smelling fresh!

WHY DOESN'T MY OWN POOP SMELL BAD TO ME?

The phrase *<name of narcissistic person> likes the smell of their own shit* comes from somewhere, and this is it. Some folks are indifferent about the smell of their defecation, while others may even like it. There's no strong scientific explanation for this besides context and familiarity—you know the poop is yours, and you're used to the odor. This more commonly applies towards farts and is why I laugh while everyone else angrily vacates the room.[66]

WHY DOES COFFEE MAKE ME GO?

People think the caffeine in coffee makes you go, but it's because it boosts gastrin levels, which is a hormone that gets things moving (acts as a laxative). So decaf coffee would work just as well if you wanted to regulate yourself but avoid caffeine. Caffeine is a diuretic, so you might also notice that you pee more too.

---

66 This is still one of my favorite activities among close family and friends. And my dog. But he does it back, so I don't feel that bad about it.

WHAT'S "BROWN FRIDAY"?

The day after Thanksgiving (commonly referred to as Black Friday) is typically when many Americans begin their early-morning Christmas shopping. But there's another cohort of people getting an early start: plumbers. Unsurprisingly, given our prior-day traditions, the day after gluttonous Thanksgiving feasting is the busiest day of the year for plumbing house calls and is known as *Brown Friday* in the home-maintenance industry—truly a time to give thanks when the family toilet stays intact.

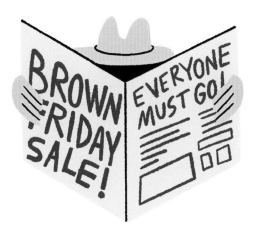

America's unofficial national holiday.

HOW DO PROFESSIONAL EATERS RECOVER AFTER A COMPETITION?

Obviously, the more you eat, the more you poop, but how does someone who is eating at a professional's scale digest everything? Well, according to participants in the Nathan's Hot Dog Eating Contest (Major League Eating's biggest competition), it can take multiple days to get rid of all the hot dogs (the world record is 76 hot dogs in 10 minutes). A key ingredient to recovery is drinking lots of water (to keep things moving) and sleeping, but not necessarily purging. The most surprising thing is that the "meat sweats" are in fact real and pretty guaranteed, so the eater's body odor smells like hot dogs. Disappointingly, but also probably for the best, professional eaters don't reveal too much about their actual stools, besides that they fill up the bowl.

HAS FLUSH TOILET DESIGN EVOLVED MUCH OVER THE YEARS?

Glad you asked! Professor Plungie, PhD in Sanitation Studies, is always ready to give a Flush History 101 lesson:

- **In the beginning:** The first-known flushing toilet was invented in ancient Rome around 31 BC by a man named Marcus Crassus. However, the technology was lost after the fall of the Roman Empire, and even at the time, most people used simple pit toilets.

- **In the Middle Ages:** Chamber pots were commonly used, and waste was often thrown out of windows into the streets. In the late Middle Ages, some castle toilets used a rudimentary form of flushing using water to wash waste away.

- **Here to stay:** The first modern flush toilet was invented by Sir John Harington in England in 1596, but it did not become widespread until the nineteenth century.

- **Innovation:** In the 1800s, the S trap was invented, which allowed for a more efficient flushing system. This was followed by the U trap, which prevented sewer gases from entering the home.

- **Advancement:** In the early 1900s, the first flush-valve toilet was invented, which allowed for a more powerful flush. In the mid-twentieth century, the first pressure-assisted toilets were introduced, which used compressed air to increase the flushing power. In the late twentieth century, low-flow toilets were introduced, which used less water and were more environmentally friendly.

- **The future is here:** In recent years, toilets with advanced features such as heated seats, automatic flushing, and built-in bidets have become more popular. Additionally, smart toilets with features such as automatic lid opening and closing, self-cleaning functions, and water-saving sensors have also been developed.

Porcelain flushable toilets have been around since the mid-nineteenth century, which is still our most common type today. Some of the flushing technology has changed, but the overall concept really hasn't that much.

WHY DO I SOMETIMES FEEL EMOTIONAL AFTER A POO SESSION?

The "Post-Poop Blues" are real, and it's quite common, especially when disposing of a rather large part of you. According to a Harvard study, we flex abdominal muscles while going, which drops our heart rate and blood pressure. This causes some folks to feel euphoric after an epic bowel movement, while others may feel temporarily sad or a bit "emptier."

PLUNGIE LIGHTNING ROUND: TOILET TRUE OR FALSE

SNAKES CAN SNEAK UP YOUR SEWER DRAIN AND INTO YOUR TOILET.

TRUE It's not common, but snakes can come up through your toilet, as well as other smaller creatures like squirrels, frogs, and rats. This is more likely to happen during warm weather. Always peek before you perch!

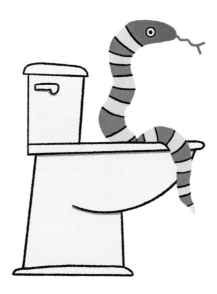

This can really happen.

THE TOILET IS THE DIRTIEST OBJECT IN YOUR HOME.

FALSE Your kitchen sink sponge, keyboard, and phone commonly have more germs on them than your toilet.[67]

PEOPLE GIVE BIRTH ON THE TOILET.

TRUE Squatting on the toilet is a very conducive position for giving birth. People sometimes accidentally give birth on the toilet without even knowing they were pregnant. So don't feel ashamed if you're a bathroom baby.

WE PICK UP THE PRESIDENT'S POOP WHEN TRAVELING ABROAD.

TRUE Stool samples have been used as counterintelligence on world leaders' health throughout history. There is a whole division to safeguard the president's poop called TOILSEC (toilet security).[68]

PEEING IN THE POOL CHANGES THE WATER COLOR.

FALSE There is no such dye in the chemical makeup of most pool water. Not endorsing the behavior of peeing in a pool, but more than likely you will get away with it. But you're not crazy: The water pressure on your kidneys does make you pee more when swimming in a pool.

---

67 However, to no surprise, the bathroom is still typically considered the smelliest room in a home.

68 Weirdly, they haven't reached out for my expert consultation services.

PEOPLE POOP IN THE MODEL TOILETS AT HOME DEPOT.

FALSE This isn't Costco, you sicko. No free sampling.

WOMEN USE MORE TOILET PAPER THAN MEN EACH YEAR.

FALSE Are you stupid? Women don't poop. But men use about 15 percent more toilet paper on average.

A GUY NAMED CRAPPER CREATED THE FLUSH TOILET.

FALSE Well, sort of. Like any origin story, it's a bit complicated. Flush toilets long existed before Thomas Crapper came along, but in the 1860s while working as a plumber in London, he created the ballcock (lol), which is a valve mechanism that prevents tank overflow. So he didn't invent the flush toilet, but he was working in the right industry at the right time to improve it in a major way and have his name historically associated with the concept!

ALMOST EVERYONE REPORTS WASHING THEIR HANDS AFTER GOING TO THE BATHROOM.

FALSE Twenty percent of people say they almost never wash their hands, but then 30 percent of the rest of the 80 percent also say they skip the soap step. So about

56 percent of the population washes their hands with soap and water. At least people are honest here, I guess.

THE "PORCELAIN PALACE" LETS UP TO A HUNDRED PEOPLE USE THE TOILET AT ONCE.

FALSE You mean the ornate complex of public toilet facilities located near the Foreigners' Street amusement park in Chongqing, China? Wow, you are so wrong. It accommodates ONE THOUSAND goers simultaneously. That toilet space is definitely not a quiet place.

IN OUR LIFETIME, WE'LL USE FOUR HUNDRED TREES' WORTH OF TOILET PAPER.

TRUE Sadly, on average, people use 384 trees' worth of toilet paper throughout their life.

TOILET PAPER USERS MAKE UP THE MAJORITY OF POOPERS.

FALSE Over four billion people still don't use it.

THE PLUNGIE PLEDGE

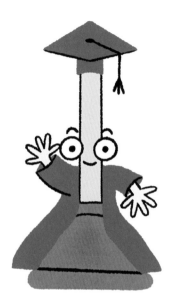

Good Toilet Citizen,

In reading this phenomenal, bestselling, life-changing book, you should now be fully trained on proper bathroom behavior and, as one might say, a *super pooper*. It is time to swear your oath of allegiance to the leader of the toilet court (naturally, that's me). This oath forbids you from ever partaking in these acts below when using the restroom. Now repeat after me:

I, _____ (your name), a student of the toilet studies, swear on this book and pledge to you, Plungie, that I will NEVER under any circumstance:

- **Knock on the bathroom door before checking if it's locked.** No need to knock if it's locked.
- **Forget to look for toilet paper before sitting down.** Empty spool means you're a fool.
- **Neglect to use a seat cover on a public toilet.** Show respect for yourself and others.
- **Repeatedly flush a clogged toilet.** You're making it worse.
- **Fail to flush.** Are you serious? What's wrong with you?
- **Leave the seat up.** Consider others.
- **Drink directly from the bathroom sink with my hands.** It makes a mess. Use a water fountain or a cup at least.
- **Procrastinate in cleaning my bathroom.** Be civilized and safe.
- **Neglect to stock enough TP.** There's no such thing as too much, but there is definitely such a thing as too little.
- **Not have any reading materials in my home bathroom.** *this book has entered the chat*

Signature: _____

You are now officially a steward of the bathroom, a leader of the loo. With great power comes great responsibility—wield it well.

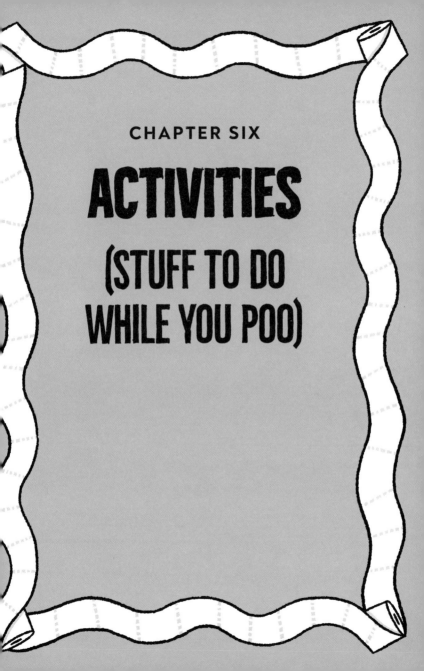

CHAPTER SIX

ACTIVITIES
(STUFF TO DO WHILE YOU POO)

Some things you can do while in the loo, besides poo. Also, some other stuff that my editor would only let me include if it was in the very back of the book, hoping you wouldn't make it that far.

(BODY) MOVEMENT FOR (BOWEL) MOVEMENT

Here are some yoga poses that you can do directly in the bathroom at home to help relieve constipation.

- **Seated Meditation:** Sit cross-legged on the closed toilet seat (if possible) or on the bathmat and focus on your breathing for five minutes. Relieving stress helps relieve bowels.
- **Forward Bend:** Keep your legs straight as you bend over and try to touch your toes. Hold this position for at least ten seconds and focus on breathing. Repeat five to ten times. This causes compression in your abdominal area, creating movement.
- **Squat Hold:** Spread your feet, keep your spine straight, and lower your butt into a deep squat. Hold for at least ten seconds and repeat five to ten times.
- **Child's Pose:** With your knees on the bath mat, slowly bend forward and try to place your palms flat

on the floor. Hold for at least ten seconds and repeat five to ten times.

- **Downward-Facing Dog:** Start by standing straight and then lean forward and put your palms onto the floor, creating a V shape with your butt lifting. Hold for at least ten seconds and repeat five to ten times. This releases traction in your spine and abdomen—great for those who sit at a desk all day (me!).

DEEP (TOILET) THOUGHTS

Don't limit your thoughts on the throne to the depth of your dunny. Like in the shower, our time on the toilet is also for pondering. Taking a seat removes some of the core distractions in life and allows the mysteries of the universe to present themselves. Here's a few deep *toilet thoughts*, but about the actual toilet.

FLUSH ATTACK: WHAT WOULD HAPPEN IF EVERYONE IN A SINGLE SEWER SYSTEM FLUSHED AT THE SAME TIME?

Let's assume all the logistical communication issues are solved. Would our sewers overflow and our collective muck emerge above ground?[69] Would flushing fail altogether? Or would everything just be totally fine?

Turns out simulations to this question have already been done, and the results are controversial. All water systems are created on a city-by-city basis, so the tipping point would happen in your local area. *Live Science* estimates that everything would probably be fine, mainly because simultaneous flushing isn't simultaneous due to each toilet being a different distance from the main sewer line. Risky bottlenecks would only build up in big apartment buildings. However, *HowStuffWorks* predicts the overflow scenario (their rough calculations were based on the city of Milwaukee, Wisconsin) and theorizes even appliances like your dishwasher could leak poopy water.[70]

What do you think will happen? Crazy answers only.

DID TOILETS INSPIRE THE DESIGN OF THE INTERNET?

The Internet is a network connecting individual devices (our phones and laptops) to a router through ethernet cable.[71] Our toilets connect to a local sewer system

---

69 Also, how does this impact the ninja turtles living down there? Would they come above ground?

70 Really good excuse to get that new kitchen set and silverware.

71 We do have wireless connections (Wi-Fi), but whatever is serving that must be physically connected by cable at some layer. No wireless toilets . . . yet. WWT (World Wide Toilets) coming soon!

through pipe plumbing. Yes, we are oversimplifying both these systems, and toilets right now only have one-way communication (HTTP is a two-way protocol—toilets only send things to the sewer system), but the basic architecture is pretty similar.

The earliest-known ideas for the Internet are accredited to Nikola Tesla at the start of the twentieth century, but weren't invented into reality until the 1960s. Designs for a flushable toilet have been around since the sixteenth century, and aqueducts were in place long before that.

So the next time you are endlessly scrolling on your phone in the bathroom, give a solid thanks to the toilet you are sitting on.

SAME SHIT, DIFFERENT DAY

The familiar phrase used to describe daily frustrations can now finally be put into practice! Go sit on your toilet just before midnight. Stay seated until the clock strikes 12:00 a.m. When finished, you literally just took the same shit but on different days.

Always let your imagination and curiosity wander to weird places when sitting on the throne; it's a judgment-free brainstorm.

ART ACTIVITY:
BUILD-A-BATHROOM

We've all seen good and bad bathrooms. Now it's time to build your ideal sanctuary, where the only limits are your imagination and sketching skills. Jacuzzis, wet bars, basketball hoops, flat-screen TVs, and tigers are all eligible in this masterpiece—let your desires wander.

Essentials required: somewhere to release, somewhere to rinse, somewhere to wash.

Dare to dream!

ART ACTIVITY:
DIY CRAFTS

Materials needed: toilet paper, fingers, folding abilities.

A practical craft is a *homemade* wet wipe, which is just a few sheets of toilet paper gently (I SAID GENTLY) rinsed under the sink to get the top layer moist. You must be precise with the wetting: too much will make your wipe break apart into crumbs.

On the other hand, toilet paper origami is an artistic craft to leave behind as a surprise for your guests to find![72] Add some décor to your sanctuary. Here are a few ideas to start:

- Flowers (classy)
- Birds (cranes are a must)
- Hearts (for the next beloved user)
- Envelopes (mail addressed to your butt)
- Shells (what do you hear if you hold it to your ear?)

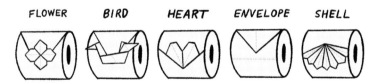

FLOWER   BIRD   HEART   ENVELOPE   SHELL

PERFECT POOPING PLAYLISTS

A pooping playlist creates a little white noise to cover up your "brown noise" and allows you to get into the zone for your session, like a pregame ritual. No matter your toilet-intended mood, this has you covered for your throne time. Go ahead and download to your device in case you're ever in offline mode while squatting. Now, here's the perfect queue for the loo. Find it here: www.playlist.ownyourthronebook.com

ANTHEMS & THEME SONGS

1. "Can't Fight This Feeling," by REO Speedwagon
2. "Should I Stay or Should I Go," by The Clash
3. "Drop It Like It's Hot," by Snoop Dogg
4. "Push It," by Salt-N-Pepa
5. "Free Fallin'," by Tom Petty
6. "Don't Stop Believin'," by Journey
7. "Let it Go," by Idina Menzel (*Frozen* soundtrack)
8. "Shake It Off," by Taylor Swift
9. "The Final Countdown," by Europe
10. "Closing Time," by Semisonic

HAPPY & HYPED

1. "Sirius," by the Alan Parsons Project (1990s Chicago Bulls warmup song)
2. "Roar," by Katy Perry
3. "All Star," by Smash Mouth

4. "Who Let the Dogs Out," by Baha Men
5. "Dancing Queen," by ABBA

SOLITUDE CELEBRATIONS

1. "Lost in My Mind," by The Head and the Heart
2. "I Think We're Alone Now," by Tiffany
3. "In My Room," by the Beach Boys
4. "Quiet Storm," by Smokey Robinson
5. "Bridge Over Troubled Water," by Simon & Garfunkel

NOT RECOMMENDED

1. "Somebody's Watching Me," by Rockwell
2. "Help!" by The Beatles
3. "Stressed Out," by Twenty One Pilots
4. "Hot in Herre," by Nelly

If you want something more instrumental, "Alexa, play rainfall" always hits the spot for some relaxing inspiration that gets things flowing. Also, anything by Hans Zimmer—the guy has proven he can score any situation beautifully.

If you want to create some privacy, I highly recommend "Halloween Theme Song," by John Carpenter (Michael Myers). Clears out a crowded bathroom every time and might even scare you into finishing up faster.

POO HAIKUS

When toilet time is a quiet solitude, it can create a moment of clarity that is highly conducive to poetry composition, especially of the 5-7-5 syllable short form, haiku. Here are a few to help inspire your own.

In a quiet place
Porcelain and water calm
Just before the splash

•••

Did the stall door lock?
Are those footsteps coming close?
An uncertain time

•••

Oh, to be at home
In my castle, on my throne
Where I reign supreme

•••

Where's the double-ply
I tire of this sandpaper
My butt needs better

•••

Blessed fuzzy seat
Plush comfort welcome and warm
This is a good day

TOILET TERMS WORD SEARCH

Quiz yourself on toilet terms with a classic word search!
Can you find them all?

D	J	M	H	S	B	I	D	E	T	C	Z	J	G
F	O	L	D	A	Y	Z	R	H	E	O	D	I	D
U	A	S	Y	L	S	G	G	H	S	U	S	F	E
V	X	H	E	O	S	S	D	F	H	R	T	A	E
S	C	R	U	N	C	H	S	P	S	T	A	C	P
P	I	L	D	E	P	O	S	I	T	E	L	I	T
F	U	S	A	H	C	D	P	Q	D	S	L	L	H
D	U	M	P	T	X	A	Y	Y	K	Y	O	I	O
M	T	P	T	C	R	H	B	W	U	F	Z	T	U
E	B	H	I	S	W	I	D	O	B	L	F	I	G
T	Z	E	R	A	Q	J	N	A	O	U	C	E	H
I	A	D	B	O	C	B	C	E	V	S	G	S	T
M	S	E	R	E	N	I	T	Y	X	H	E	K	S
E	L	U	Z	S	B	E	C	R	A	P	P	E	R

ALONE	DEEP THOUGHTS	LATRINE
BIDET	DEPOSIT	ME TIME
CABOOSE	DUMP	SERENITY
COURTESY FLUSH	FACILITIES	STALL
CRAPPER	FOLD	THRONE

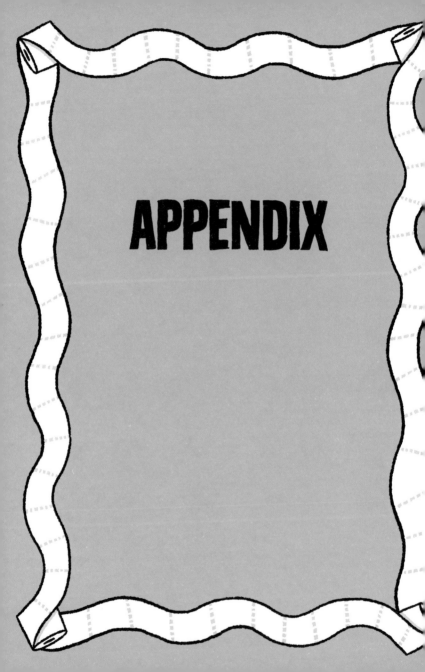

APPENDIX

USEFUL EUPHEMISMS

Go crazy creatively with some of these more obscure (but valid) toilet terms!

BUTT

back office

badonkadonk

bahootie

bottom

breeches

bum-fiddle

buns

caboose

cake

can

cheeks

donk

double jugs

duff

dump truck

dumper

fanny

fart box

full moon

heinie

hindquarters

hunkers

money maker

rump

seat cushion

sit-upon

sitzfleisch

stern

trunk

tuchus

turd cutter

tushie

wagger

TOILET

bogger

brasco

cloakroom

comfort station

commode

convenience

docking station

dunny

facilities

poop pipes

poop shoot

porcelain throne

pot

release seat

sewer seat

spicy cauldron

spin master

stain drain

turd tub

turd tube

wastebasket

water closet

whirlpool

POOPING

back ending

bark parking

bookkeeping

bowl bombing

brick laying

building a log
cabin

butt cutting

crock-potting
potatoes

cutting rope

downsizing

dropping

entry logging

floating a trout

freeing the turtles

launching a butt
shuttle

pipe laying

planting a tree

reigning supreme

releasing the
kraken

shedding skin

taking out the
trash

torpedo shooting

underwater
sculpting

unloosing the
caboose

waste management

working through
your backlog

CELEBRATE WORLD TOILET DAY (NOVEMBER 19TH)

Give some gratitude to that special shitter in your life because we totally take for granted that we even have access to one.[73] It's perhaps not a coincidence that the holiday takes place a week before Thanksgiving, which is the American bathroom community's busiest shift of the year. Like bringing your mom breakfast in bed every Mother's Day, make a point each November to give your toilet a fresh scrub of gratefulness for all the waste discarding that year.

But in all seriousness, this holiday was created in 2013 to inspire and create awareness around the fact that *over three billion people still don't have safely managed sanitation*[74] (nearly half the earth's population) and half a billion still practice open defecation. This can cause feces to contaminate primary drinking-water sources, which leads to illness, disease, and even death. It blows my privileged mind that I've written a whole book about something so core to my everyday routine, yet many folks still have never flushed a toilet. If you would like to learn more about this cause or help contribute, please visit www.worldtoiletday.info.

---

73 I would be in serious trouble without my toilet.
74 This means basic sanitation services where waste is disposed off-site and safely. Basically, a sewer system that handles all waste for a region.

A TOILET-TIME RHYME

Well, what have we learned?
Let's recap in a rhyme,
And just like this book,
It's about toilet time.

Preparation is key,
By now you should know,
When we set out to find,
The best place to go.

Public potties may vary,
Each with minus and plus,
Choose carefully in need,
To dodge bother and muss.

As you find yourself walking,
Into a dear stall,
Do your best to secure,
Its firm entrance wall.

Before setting in,
There's one crucial thing,
Check for toilet paper,
If you did not bring.

On the job do not fret,
When you must go at work,
You're being paid for this time (hopefully),
Gladly squat with a smirk.

For your comfort at home,
Trick out the throne room,
Add soft candles and plush,
Padded seats and perfume.

Considerate user, be,
Of this sacred shared space,
When you've finished your business,
Try to leave not a trace.

When finally finished,
With the bowl now to spin,
Mind you—first close the lid,
Keep particles within.

Well at last, dear reader,
Our journey's end is near,
May your toilet career,
Flush with joy, never fear!

SOME EMERGENCY TOILET PAPER PAGES

In case of a no-toilet-paper emergency, tear out and use these pages.[75]

---

75 This book is printed on uncoated paper. You are welcome. Dispose in a trash receptacle. Do not flush.

Emergency toilet paper

ACKNOWLEDGMENTS

I want to thank Steve Mockus at Chronicle Books, for hearing some of my more "unconventional" ideas, and Kirsten Janene-Nelson, for helping craft this concept in its very initial stages.

To Laura Mazer at Wendy Sherman Associates, for representing my vision for this project and introducing me to the fundamentals of publishing.

To all my friends, for sharing their own toilet thoughts and troubles, especially some named Allen (the formula master), Bradley, Dirty Mike (the throne trailblazer), and Trevor.

And finally, thank you, dear reader, for sticking around to this point. I hope you continue to make every throne feel like your very own.

Assuming you're now finished with this book, spread the loo love and leave this copy in a random bathroom for the next goer to find. This is the one acceptable time to break the Leave No Trace philosophy!

ABOUT THE AUTHOR

Bradford Ware lives in New York City, and has a tiny head with a big body. In his spare time outside the bathroom he loves sitting in saunas, admiring bonsai trees, and producing eccentric animations under the alias Elderly Boy Studios. This is his first book, which was written from a toilet in Oakland, California.

ABOUT THE ILLUSTRATOR

Em Spitler is an art director, illustrator, and artist whose work has been recognized with many awards (including the ADDYs, PRINT Awards, American Graphic Design Awards, the Art Directors Club Awards, and Pentawards), and whose illustrations have appeared in CDC campaigns, *Whalebone* magazine features, collaborative projects with Sightglass Coffee, and interactive NYC pop-ups.

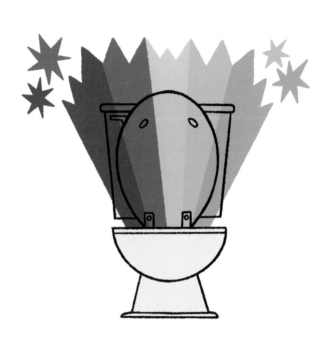